# THE NEW YOU

W. Marshall Guy, MD

# A Physician's Pledge

Simply by reading this book you have taken the first step to using time-tested ways to improve your appearance. This book helps to dispel many of the myths and caution against the "to-good-to-be-true" procedures that exist in facial rejuvenation. Furthermore, it helps you to understand why an individualized plan including surgical and non-surgical options can prove to be the most beneficial and cost-effective measure to help you restore and maintain your youthful appearance. Throughout this book you will be provided with information that gives you the insight you need to ask better questions and make more informed decisions. You will also be able to learn about what to expect before, during, and after procedures with clearly delineated instructions that, when followed, provided the best opportunity to achieve the desired results.

As you learn about the different options, it should become clear that your plan will be customized to you as opposed to a "one-size-fits-all" approach. Each procedure is carefully planned to provide you with the greatest improvement with the least amount of risk. At the same time great care is taken to avoid the "overdone" or "plastic" look. The goal is to always create a very natural appearance. This is achieved by using time tested techniques refined to provide you with the result you want. It is important to realize that new is not always better when it comes to fads in plastic surgery, and that by using tried and true techniques we can help to achieve our mutual goals.

When I became a physician, I pledged an oath to apply my knowledge for your benefit, to avoid overtreatment and refrain from treatment that doesn't help. From that oath I will recommend not only treatments that are designed to improve your appearance but also all aspects of your health and life. And, if you grant me the opportunity to become your surgeon, that's exactly what I will do.

I, along with my staff, are honored that you have taken this first step towards the new you. When we meet at the time of your consultation, I will recommend the procedures, products, and treatments that will provide you with the greatest result at your particular stage of life. Although I can never guarantee results, there is one promise I can make: I will do everything to the best of my ability and within my power to justify the trust you have provided in me and to make your experience as pleasant as possible.

W. Marshall Guy, MD

## Preface

The book you hold before you is called "The New You." This particular title was decided upon after much deliberation. The reason this title has been chosen is because regardless of whether you undergo any treatment, you have already taken a step towards improving your life. The knowledge you will gain from these pages will make you a more informed consumer, able to better participate in your health, and ready to lead a healthier life.

It is recommended that you read the first three (3) chapters regardless of what procedure(s) you are interested in as they provide very useful information. In addition, you should read chapter 13 about scar revision and the wound healing process. After reading these chapters, please read the specific chapters on the procedure(s) you are interested in being evaluated for prior to your consultation.

## Acknowledgements

This book is adapted in part with permission from E. Gaylon McCollough's "The Appearance Factor." As a mentor and fellowship director, it was with his training and tutelage that has allowed me to fulfill my dream. In addition, the training I received from my co-fellowship director, Dr. Fred Fedok has been invaluable. As both of these men have been former presidents of the American Academy of Facial Plastic & Reconstructive Surgery, the training I received was world class.

I would also like to thank the many talented facial plastic surgeons of whom I have had the experience of training and working with including Anthony E. Brissett MD, Krista Olson MD, Eugene Alford MD, and Russell Kridel MD.

# About the Author

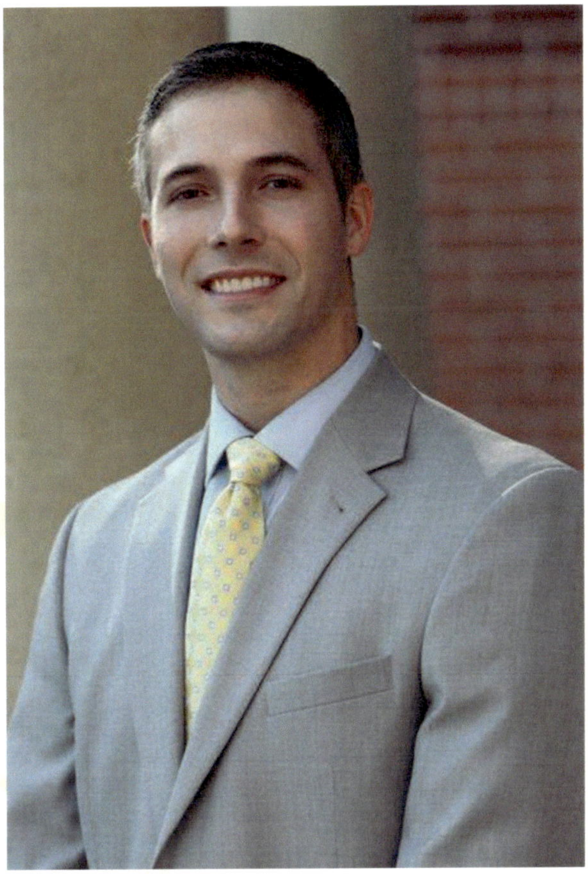

Dr. Guy grew up in the Spring-Klein area. He attended St. Thomas High School where he was captain of two varsity sports and was the highest-ranking graduate at this prestigious college preparatory school. He received his undergraduate education at the University of Texas at Austin where he was selected as a member of the natural sciences honors program known as the Dean's scholars. He also received many academic based scholarships. He graduated with highest honors with a 4.0 GPA with a major in biology and a minor in Spanish. He attended Baylor College of Medicine in the heart of the Texas Medical Center for medical school where he graduated with highest honors (highest ranking graduate). He also received multiple honors and awards including election into both the Alpha Omega Alpha Medical Honor Society (based on academic excellence) and the Gold Humanism Honor Society (based on his demonstration of the qualities of integrity, excellence, compassion, altruism, respect, and empathy). He stayed in Houston where he attended one of the most sought-after residency programs in the country at Baylor College of Medicine in Otolaryngology-Head and Neck Surgery. This is where he learned the intricacies of the structures of the neck, face, and nose working at such facilities including Houston Methodist Hospital, MD Anderson Cancer Center, Ben Taub General Hospital, Texas Children's Hospital, St. Lukes Hospital, and the Michael E. Debakey Veteran's Administration Hospital.

Dr. Guy continued to excel in residency and was selected to attend the prestigious Facial Plastic Surgery Fellowship under the world renowned Facial Plastic Surgeons, Drs. E. Gaylon McCollough and Fred Fedok. It is here where he continued to refine his surgical skills in the art of facial rejuvenation and reconstructive surgery under tutelage from the field's masters.

Dr. Guy returned to the Houston area and The Woodlands at the completion of his fellowship to open his own practice as a double board certified, fellowship trained, facial plastic surgeon. Dr. Guy has strived for excellence throughout his life, and he looks forward to using his knowledge and skills to help you look your best.

# Table of Contents

# Chapter 1

## An Introduction to Cosmetic Plastic Surgery

**How Much is Beauty Worth at Work**

**Philosophy**

**Before and After**

**Individualized Care**

**The Aging Face**

**Surgery for the Aging Face**

**The Antidote to "One-Size-Fits-All" Surgery**

# How Much Is Beauty Worth at Work?

On July 8, 2010 Newsweek published the results of two polls it had conducted of 202 hiring managers at corporate organizations, ranging from human-resources employees to senior-level vice presidents. It also included a telephone survey of 964 members of the public to verify what no one wants to admit: that in all elements of the workplace, looks matter, and they matter greatly. The 8 most interesting revelations of this poll include:

1. **Looks Do Matter At Work**
   Almost 60% of managers believe that an unattractive but equally qualified applicant will have a harder time getting hired, and two-thirds believe that even once hired, looks will continue to affect the ratings given for job performance. The survey from the general public provided similar ratings.

2. **Looks Matter More than Education, Apparently**
   When asked to rank 10 applicant qualities from 1 the least important and 10 the greatest, looks came in at 7.1. This was third behind experience and confidence but above where the applicants went to school. This is not to say you should forego an education and use the money on cosmetic surgery, but it does show that not everyone is looking for an Ivy League Diploma

3. **Put Your Money Where Your Mouth Is. (We Suppose That Could Be taken Literally.)**
   Fifty-nine percent of hiring managers advised applicants to spend as much time making sure they look attractive as on perfecting their résumés.

4. **Yes, We Knew This: It's Worse for Women**
   As a whole, women are perceived to benefit more from their looks than men, but this also puts more pressure on women. Almost 40% of the managers believed that being "very good-looking" is more of an advantage for women than men.

5. **Hiring Mangers Discriminate Against Overweight Applicants**
   Despite the fact that almost 75% of Americans are considered overweight, two thirds of business managers said they believe some managers would hesitate before hiring a qualified applicant who was significantly overweight.

6. **Managers Also Dislike Old People**
   Eight-four percent of managers said they believe some bosses would hesitate hiring a qualified applicant who looked significantly older than his peers.

7. **Hiring Based On Looks Is OK. (In Certain Situations).**
   Nearly two-thirds of hiring managers said they believe companies should be allowed to hire based on looks when the employee is to be the "face" of a company.

8. **Confidence Is Important, Too!**
   Both confidence and experience ranked higher on the list of most important employee attributes.

In further support of the *Newsweek* survey, it is apparent that when one looks one's best, self-confidence improves. Therefore, improving one's looks can also help to bolster other hiring factors.

## Philosophy

Your appearance matters in society. This is not just a statement but a fact. Research has shown more attractive people earn more money, are more likely to be hired and promoted, and are more likely to draw in customers when all things are considered. Furthermore, more attractive people are often judged to be more kind, decent, and honest. Even the renowned philosopher, Aristotle, commented that, "Beauty is a greater recommendation than any letter of introduction." Considering how many doors the right letter of recommendation could open, this "secret" to successful living should be taken seriously by anyone committed to creating a memorable impression. And, although the definition of beauty changes with time, numerous experts have supported the finding that favors are granted to people considered to be attractive.

I am a firm believer that inner beauty and physical beauty are complementary and that improving one will improve the other. As you begin this journey of rejuvenation and take the steps to improve your physical appearance you will improve your mental wellbeing as well. One of the best ways to naturally improve your mental self is with exercise. This is not coincidental as the body releases endorphins with exercise which are one of the chemicals in the body that makes you feel good. At the same time, as your health improves you have more energy, and you feel better about how you look and about yourself. James Allen, who may well be the precursor of all self-help authors, wrote, "The body is the servant of the mind." It is only once the mind realizes the beauty you have that you can truly feel youthful. As one improves, so will the other. Cosmetic surgery is a complementary part of the process of rejuvenation. By improving the signs of aging, you can look as good on the outside as you feel on the inside.

And although everyone is not born with the perfect proportions of attractiveness, there are certain learned behaviors and actions that can improve one's overall "appeal." This includes how you carry yourself, how you stand without slouching, and how you sit. Your overall level of physical fitness can improve your appeal. How you coordinate your attire including clothes and accessories affects the impression you create. Finally, your outlook on life, how cheerful you are towards others, and letting your inner beauty shine through can improve your appeal. These are all attributes which can be improved without any surgical intervention which is why there is virtually no excuse for not looking one's best.

For those patients who are appropriate surgical candidates and desire to maximize his or her appeal, the right surgical procedure performed by the right surgeon for the right reasons can play a vital role regardless of age.

For individuals just beginning to shows the signs of aging, "maintenance surgery" can go a long way to preserve your youthful appearance. For those with more advanced signs of aging, an experienced surgeon can restore the body to a more youthful appearance. I take a very natural approach to surgery. Through my extensive training in facial plastic and reconstructive surgery, I can create a very natural, refreshed look and avoid the "operated on" look, as you can see in the before and after section. Age truly is just a number, and there is never a better time to look your best. Schedule a consultation today because you deserve it!

## Before and After

The next several pages demonstrate pre and post-operative results of patients who underwent a variety of procedures covered in this book including what they had to say about Dr. Guy. All of the procedures demonstrated here were personally performed by Dr. Guy. All photographs in this book are used to demonstrate the result obtained in that particular case and should not be used for comparison or as a guarantee of future results.

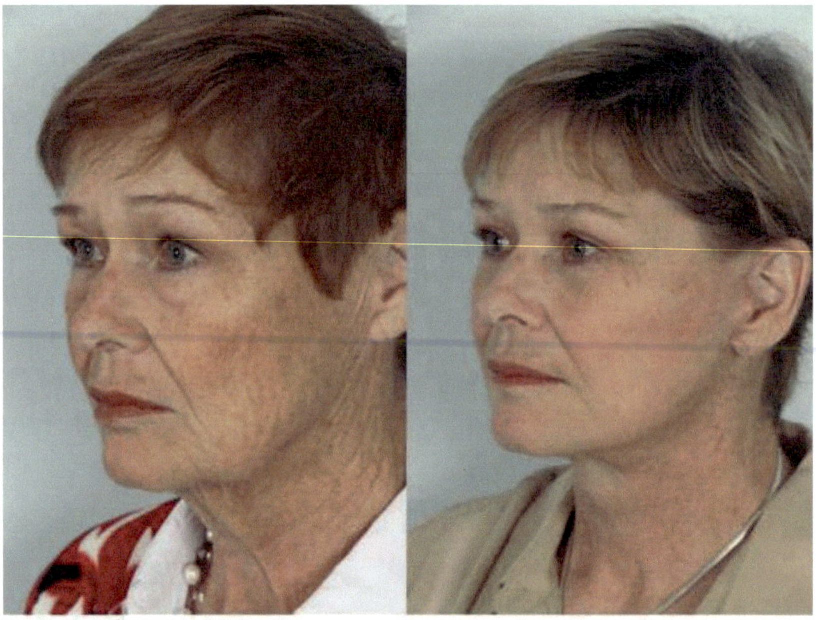

Before DR. GUY FACIAL PLASTIC SURGERY After

"This is the only review you will have to read about Dr. W. Marshall Guy. Put your trust in all I have to say about this extraordinary person and incredible doctor. I will start off by asking the question, "Why does one choose to have facial plastic surgery"? After all it is an elective surgery and a costly one too. It is scary and by all means frightening or at least in my case I will say it was. It's all about the unknown. What if it doesn't go right? What if I do not look like myself. What if I am pulled to tight? The unknowns go on and on. You have chosen to have this operation all in the name of "vanity". This is my experience and why I would do it again without a moment's hesitation if Dr. Guy were my plastic surgeon. I literally woke up one morning and said to myself you are going to call the McCollough Institute today and schedule a consultation with Dr. McCollough. I went in, had the consultation, and I was put on the books for surgery September 23, 2014. I had made my decision. If I were going to have plastic surgery it was going to be at the McCollough Institute. A few weeks later I got a call from the clinic saying my surgery had to be rescheduled until the 8th of January, 2015. I was disappointed but in life I realize things always work out for the best. I was not supposed to have surgery on Sept. 23. On January 8th I am at the clinic at 6:00am. I have not met my doctor yet.

At the last moment I chose to have a fellow perform my surgery. When I walked in the clinic my doctor, Dr. Guy, was standing at the end of the hall waiting for me to arrive. He walked over to me and took my hand and patted it and said I am going to take the best care of you that I can. At the moment I knew I could put all my trust in him and let go of my fears. He had that aura surrounding him and my instincts never fail me. I knew I was in good hands. Dr. Guy is the epitome of a surgeon. He is at the top of plastic surgeons and there he will always remain. The care, the devotion and self-drive of this amazing person will never waiver. Dr. Guy becomes very connected to you as a patient. He cares, he truly listens, and is thorough in his approach to caring for you. There is no question left unanswered. He wants your recovery and healing process to be stress free. He goes "over the top" to do just that. If you're happy then he has done his job. He takes every step of the journey with you. He makes sure you fully understand all aspects of the healing process. You have his cell number. Your calls and text are followed up with prompt attention. Dr. Guy's character, integrity, and professionalism is unsurpassed. If you are contemplating cosmetic surgery there is only one very special doctor to consider and that is Dr. W. Marshall Guy. Period end! He will deliver, in that I promise!"

This patient is 3 months out from her facelift that involved her cheek, neck, and temporal area. Two days after her surgery she also underwent a full-face resurfacing with a fractionated carbon dioxide laser. Notice the overall improvement in her skin quality and jaw line. Even from this oblique view you can see the neck improvement. You can see the improvement in the fullness over her cheekbones and the improvement in the hollowness below her cheek as a result of repositioning her own tissue back to where it was when she was younger. It's also important to notice you cannot see any of her incisions as I place them in locations that helps them stay camouflaged.

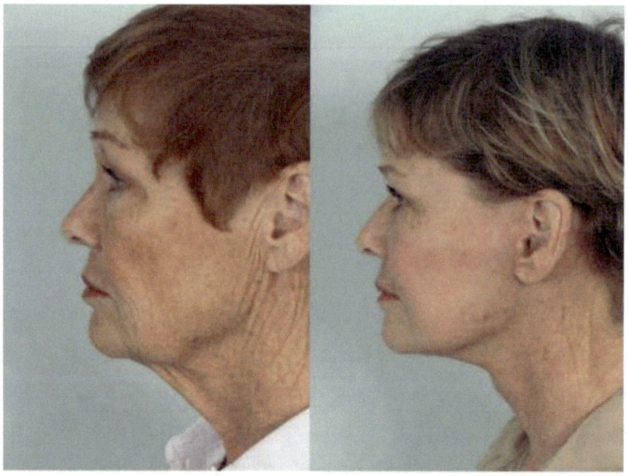

Before DR. GUY FACIAL PLASTIC SURGERY After

This is the same patient from above but from a profile view. You can see the significant improvement in her neck and jowls as well as the texture of her skin.

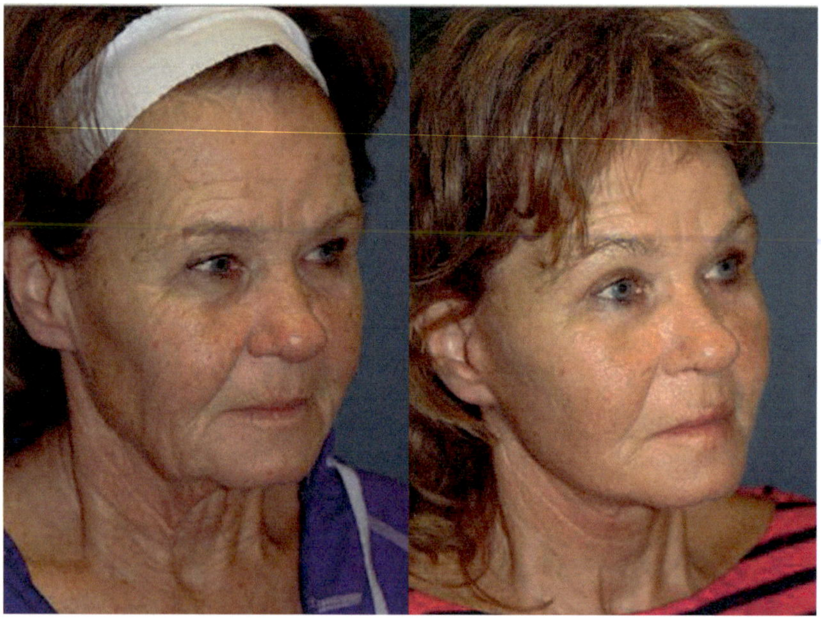

"I had surgery in February of 2015 and had a total face procedure. Even though I was nervous about surgery I was not nervous about having Dr Guy as my surgeon. He made me confident in the process of healing and I am pleased with what he performed on me. I don't look like I had surgery. I look like myself, just minus the sagging signs of age. He just brought out what I look like before things started to breakdown on my appearance. I really appreciate his talent and appreciate him. He pays attention to detail and is a very talented doctor. I'm glad I met him."

This patient in her 50s is 11 weeks out following a full facelift including the forehead, temple, cheek, and neck areas. In addition, she had an upper and lower blepharoplasty plus upper and lower lip augmentation and advancement. She notes that she looked at a picture from her 30s and following her surgery she looks the same. You will frequently hear me say the goal of surgery is to restore you to how you looked 12-15 years ago, and this patient did that and more. Yet, nothing about her looks "done," which is the natural look that I strive to create for you. You can see how the hollowness in her cheeks seen in the picture above has been replaced with the soft tissue that had sunken down to create her jowls. The sagging skin of her neck is now rejuvenated all the way down to her collarbone. You can see the overall improvement in her appearance from her eyebrows down to her neck. You can see how much her neck has improved. What you don't see are her incisions as I planned them to be in natural transitions of her face. As you can expect, this patient was ecstatic with her result.

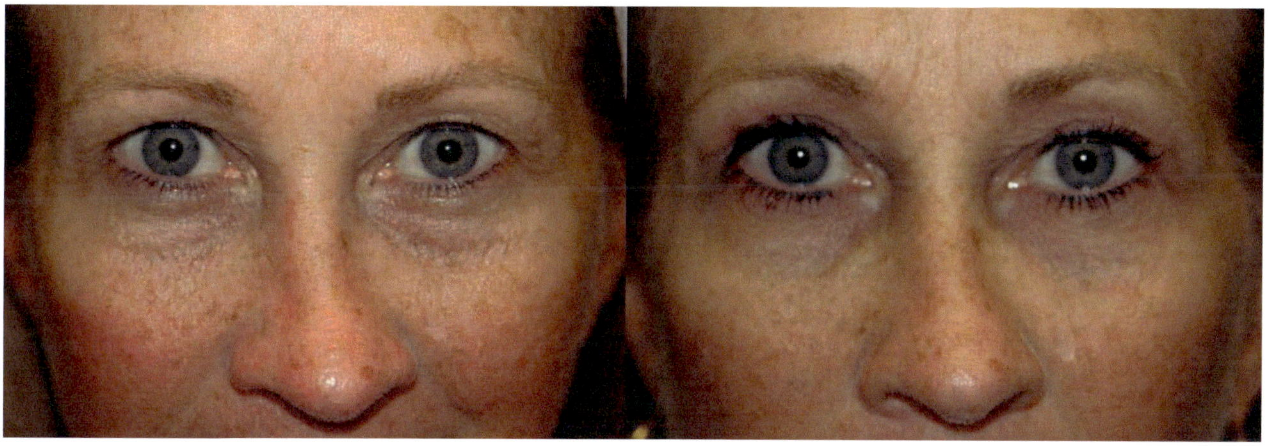

This patient in her 50s is 2 weeks out following an upper eyelid blepharoplasty performed under local anesthesia in the clinic. You can see her lack of swelling and bruising. In fact, most people would not be able to tell she had had surgery only two weeks ago. Notice the improvement in the eyelid skin and how it no longer hangs over her eyelashes. In fact, in the after photo you can see her upper eyelid eyelashes which were nearly completely hidden in the before photo.

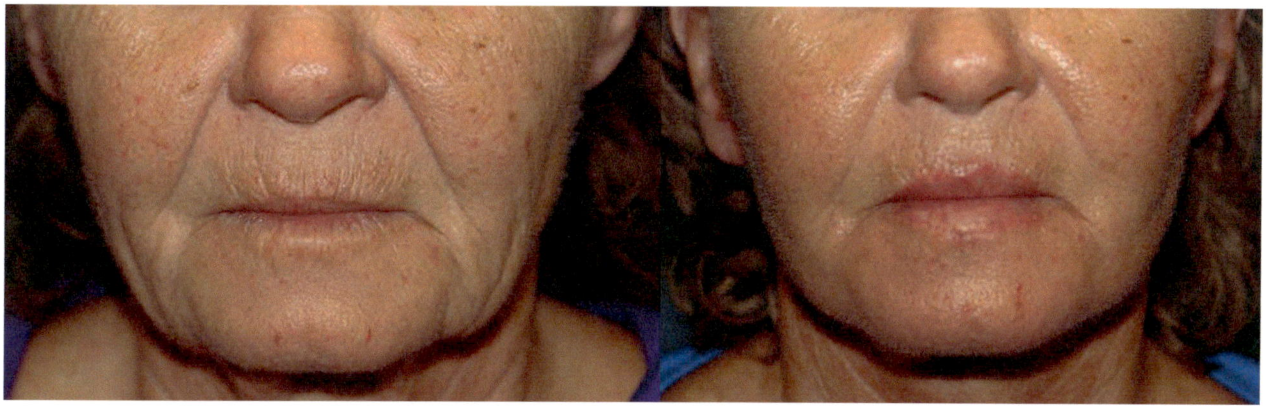

This patient is 12 weeks after undergoing lip enhancement. She had both a lip advancement procedure as well as lip augmentation using her own collagen at the time of her face lift. Note the rejuvenation she has had around her mouth and lips. The lip advancement allows more of her red lip to show, reversing one of the tell-tale signs of aging. The lip augmentation procedure complemented the lip advancement by providing greater fullness to her lips, a sign of youth.

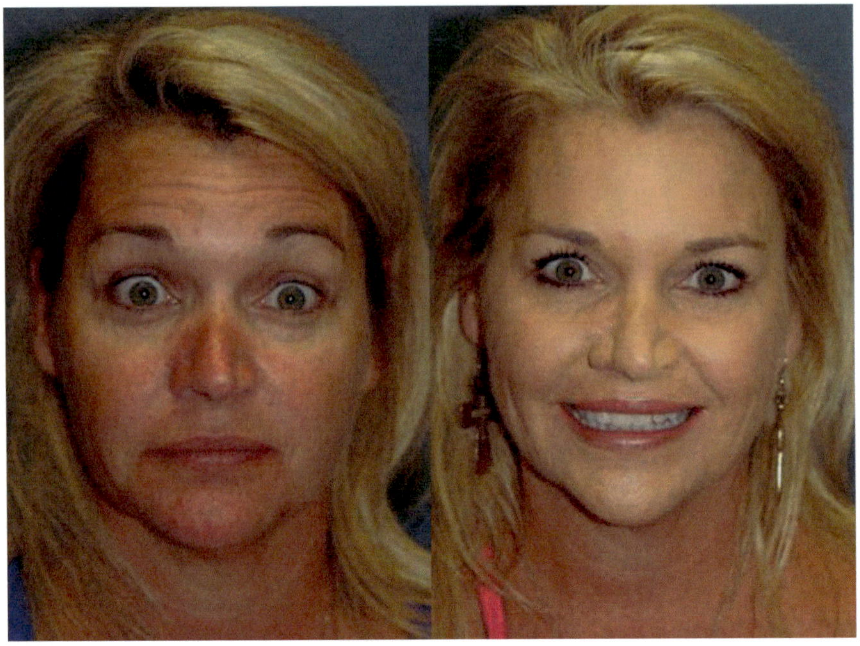

"Love him!!!!!!! My results are fantastic. I would highly recommend him. Dr Guy explained everything before he got started and during procedure I was at ease."

This patient is 1 week post treatment with 10 units of Botox to her forehead, 20 units of Botox to her glabella (vertical 1s) and 10 units of Botox to each lateral periorbital rhytids (Crow's feet). Notice with activity how there are no longer any active wrinkles in those areas. In the after you can tell she is trying to exert motion as she is opening her eyes much wider than at rest. Also note that there is no drooping of her eyebrows or eyelids with the techniques I use. The camera flash was not working properly at the before photo which is the only reason a flash was used after and not before. No attempt has been made to artificially improve the photo with the use of a post procedural flash.

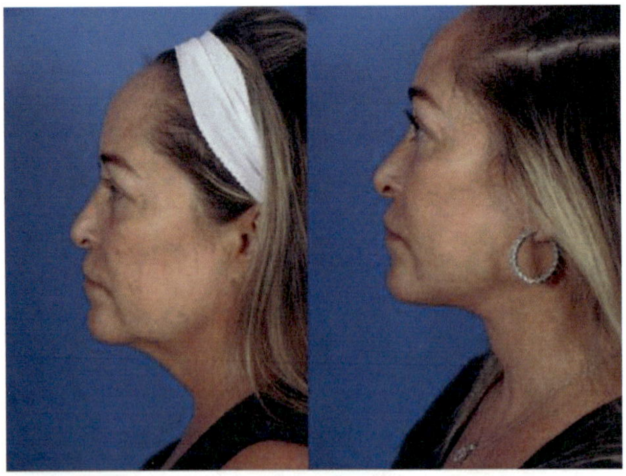

Before DR. GUY Facial Plastic Surgery After

This patient in her 50s is 8 months out from her facelift and lower eyelid surgery. From this view you can see the improvement she had in her neck and jawline. Her biggest concerns before surgery was the heaviness of her neck and jowls. In the after photo you can see how her neck has a nice defined angle and the jawline is now smooth instead of hanging.

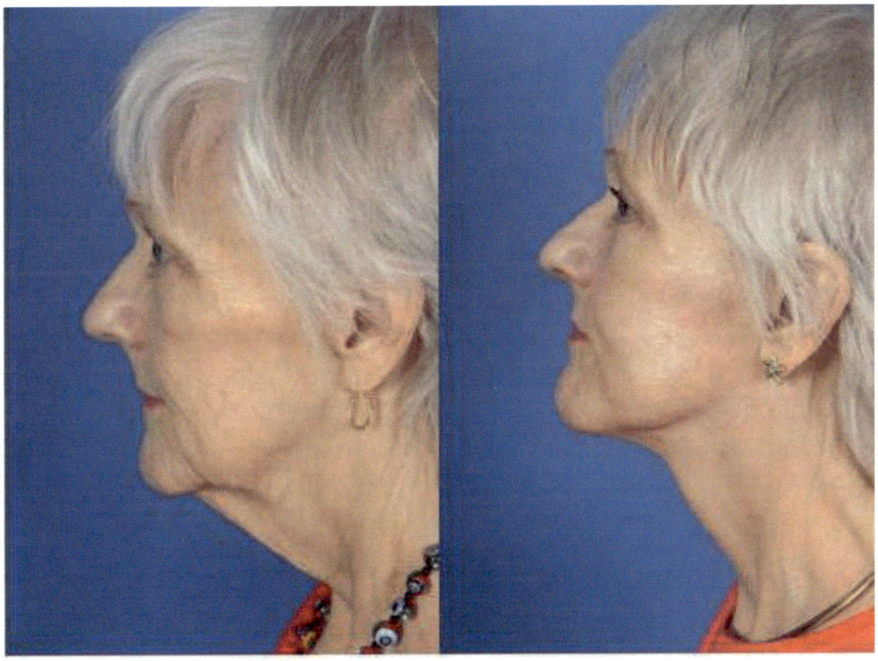

Before DR. GUY FACIAL PLASTIC SURGERY After

This patient in her 70s is 8 months out from her deep plane cheek and neck lift with Dr. Guy. Notice the improved jawline and neck line but still a natural, non-operated look.

## Individualized Care

These cases demonstrate what can be achieved when patients have realistic expectations and follow the instructions both before and after treatment. At your time of consultation, we will develop an *individualized* treatment plan based on your wishes and budget.

Although it is possible to undergo "extreme" makeovers, the majority of patients who undergo consultation are interested in *maintaining* their youthful appearance or enhancing only those areas of greatest concern. During your consultation, you will have the opportunity to express your concerns and desires and have your questions answered. If you are a candidate for surgery, based on the goals we have set we can do as much or as little as you want to have done either at one time or staged over several surgeries. You are the boss!

## The Aging Face

The face ages in a natural progression. Some people age sooner, others more slowly. Some age faster in one area of the face and maintain youth in others. However, in general there are trends that can be seen.

Beginning in the mid to late thirties you will see the outside of the eyebrows, the cheeks, and the neck begin to descend slightly. This process continues and commonly leads to a "frowning" or "tired" look. With the greater descent of these tissues with further age you begin to notice a series of ridges and hollows developing where the ridge used to fill in the hollow above it. The folds around the mouth become more prominent. The jowls begin to hang down below the jaw and the jawline begins to blend with the neck. A pocket of adipose (fat) tissue begins to develop below the chin creating a wattle. The muscle that used to support the neck weakens and can form bands running from the chin to the sternum (breast bone). The tip of the nose begins to drop as its supporting structures weaken which can lead to the appearance of a hump. The lips begin to thin, especially the upper. The area between the nose and mouth gets longer and the pink part of the upper lip begins to turn towards the teeth and can even disappear. The skin begins to show wrinkles with animation. This progresses from wrinkles with motion to wrinkles noticeable at rest. Sun damage takes its toll and shows uneven skin tones, pigmented spots, and in some circumstances precancerous lesions. The earlobes continue to lengthen and thin and the hair thins and can recede. All of this progresses until you exhibit the undesirable characteristics of "old age."

But it is possible to prevent and correct many of these signs of aging through both proactive skin care and a "youthful maintenance surgery approach," so you give the appearance that you never seem to age. The other approach is the retrospective or after the fact approach to aging. This addresses the signs of aging after they have occurred. Both approaches are effective, and the bottom line is that surgery is available either to retain or regain a youthful appearance.

One of the dilemmas facing consumers is how to find the right surgeon to perform the right operation(s). To ensure that patients do not pay for more surgery than is needed, the cost of each procedure is adjusted by the amount of surgery performed. For the younger patient looking to maintain the youthful appearance the procedure required is less extensive so it would not be as expensive when compared to the patient who waits until more advanced aging is present.

## Surgery for the Aging Face

Surgery that addresses facial aging must focus on more than sagging skin of the cheeks and neck. While a "face lift" is frequently part of the surgical plan, other options may be considered depending on the signs of aging. Many patients will benefit from work on the eyebrows and eyelids to remove bags in those regions and make the eyes appear more rested and open. Those with sun damaged skin may consider skin resurfacing procedures. Liposuction may be added to those who need it to better contour the face and neck. It is important to realize that a number of "accessorizing procedures" can be carried out at the same time as a face lift without adding time to the overall recovery.

In order to maintain or recapture a youthful appearance, not all faces should have the same treatment. Facial rejuvenation plans ought to be personalized to meet the goals and desires of each patient. But we live in a world of instant gratification with heavy marketing and commercialization of this industry. It is often this commercialization for the "latest and greatest" that drives consumers instead of verifiable science to support claims. Many physicians respond by giving patients what they ask for instead of what they need. The danger in this trend is that corporate executives instead of physicians begin to guide medical therapy. And today's fad becomes tomorrow's complication.

## The Antidote to "One-Size-Fits-All" Surgery

With a rise in commercialization of cosmetic surgery, the public becomes inundated with "franchised" procedures which represent little more than a catchy title. Others still utilize the term "face lift" despite not involving any surgical tightening or removing of excess, loose skin. This isn't to say that some of these techniques don't have their uses. But their misleading labeling and attempts to direct all patients towards the "one-size-fits-all" treatment is concerning, as this fails to create the kinds of results that could be obtained by a surgeon skilled in a variety of rejuvenating techniques. It is based on the time-tested and scientifically verified surgical approaches that I practice which help to provide not only the best option for you but also the one designed to provide the longest result without appearing "overdone." These can be combined with other adjunctive therapies such as fillers, neuromodulators, and quality skin care to provide the unified treatment goal of helping to restore a youthful appearance.

# Chapter 2

## Preparing for your Consultation

**Informed Consent and Risks**

**Self-Analysis: The Home Mirror Check-Up**

*Facial Analysis*

**The Consultation: Conferring with Dr. Guy**

**Consultation Fees**

**Scheduling Your Surgery**

**The Costs of Surgery**

**Operating Room and Facility Fees**

**Laboratory and Medical Work Up**

**Developing a Long-Term Doctor-Patient Relationship**

## Informed Consent and Risks

The ultimate decision to undergo elective surgery resides with you, the patient. It is important to have support from those around you including family and friends. However, the final decision is ultimately yours.

- Every patient is not a good candidate for surgery nor is surgery recommended for everyone who comes in because it may not be the best option at this time. When other options are more appropriate such as energy devices like EmbraceRF, neuromodulators, or fillers these will be discussed. The same holds true if these other modalities would be of benefit for your individualized rejuvenation plan. Before proceeding with any surgery, several facts need to be both understood and accepted:
- First, the goal of any operation should be improvement and not perfection. If you expect perfection, then you should not undergo cosmetic surgery as this is almost never attainable.
- Second, the degree of success of the operation depends not only on the skill of your surgeon but also on your age, overall health, skin quality, underlying bone structure, other medical problems, expectations, and the imponderables of the healing process, some of which can be aided and some of which is based on your innate ability to heal.
- Third, the motives which direct you towards cosmetic surgery should be realistic. Surgery is not a cure all for life's problems. The resulting cosmetic improvement may be psychologically beneficial as a result of increased self-esteem. However, if you blame your appearance for the lack of success or happiness in life, then surgery should not be undertaken. It is also possible that the wishes of the patient are surgically unattainable or inadvisable.
- Fourth, while most facial procedures carry minimal pain and discomfort, you must be prepared to accept the pain with the assistance of pain medication provided by your surgeon.
- Fifth, every surgical procedure entails risk both in terms of serious complications and the possibility that it may not match your expectations. Some of the risks associated with surgery may include but are not limited to: reactions to anesthesia or other medical preparations, poor wound healing, injuries to muscles and nerves, numbness, swelling, skin discoloration, facial distortion, asymmetries, excessive scarring, and many others including those statistically unlikely such as blindness, paralysis, heart attack, stroke, or even death. Although complications rarely occur, patients are encouraged to inquire further about the risks of the surgery they are contemplating.
- Sixth, it would be unethical for any physician to guarantee results. Therefore, I cannot guarantee an outcome from any treatment, but I do strive to do my best to help you achieve your realistic goals.
- Seventh, some degree of swelling occurs after any surgical procedure. This is a result of the body bringing new fluid into the area to promote healing. The increased blood supply is responsible for the pink color of the skin that is sometimes confused with discoloration after surgery. As the body heals and the fluid is not needed, it is absorbed back into

the blood stream. It is very common for the fluid to go away faster on one side or for it to collect in one area. This can lead to the sensation of lumps and bumps. Most of these, if not all, will disappear as tissues heal. Sometimes steroid injections can speed the healing process.

- Eighth, when an incision is made that is the entire thickness of the skin it will heal by producing a scar. Using plastic surgery techniques, attempts are made to keep scars narrow and camouflaged in natural facial folds and creases or hidden by the hairline. During this healing process the initial scar will be pink and somewhat swollen and lumpy. They will usually become less conspicuous as the healing process continues, up to a year or longer in younger patients. Failure to absolutely adhere to the postoperative instructions can cause scars to widen and/or thicken. Because pulling on a scar will cause it to widen and thicken, be prepared to limit physical activity for a while after surgery.
- Ninth, no matter how skillfully the skin and underlying tissues are drawn during surgery, in time they will loosen. It is impossible to predict when and to what extent this will happen. Genetics, age differences, stress, illness, nicotine use, sun exposure, nutrition, etc., all play a role in how soon a "tuck-up" procedure may be considered.
- Finally, your overall attitude, health, and adherence to the staff's instructions play an important role in the results of any surgery. It is a must that you inform us of any medical conditions you have, medications you take (including herbal remedies and over-the-counter medications), allergies, and any complications you may have experienced with previous surgery. Prior to any procedure requiring anesthesia, a check-up from your primary care physician with surgical clearance provided by this physician is required. Depending on your medical conditions, other specialists' clearance may be required.

## Self-Analysis: The Home Mirror Check-Up

A series of photographs will be obtained at your consultation to assist in planning your surgery. Prior to coming to the clinic, you should analyze yourself in front of a mirror using the below criteria.

**Facial Analysis:**

It is rare to see a face that is perfectly symmetrical. It is much more common to have differences between the two sides of the face. For example, one eyebrow, nostril, or corner of the mouth might be higher than the other. One ear, cheek, or part of the chin may project more than its counterpart. This is pointed out not to alarm you but rather to show you that minor differences in facial structures are considered perfectly normal. It is important to know about them before surgery because after surgery most people begin to really analyze their face and would be alarmed if they weren't aware about the differences ahead of time. Some of these asymmetries can be improved with surgery while others cannot.

Based on descriptions from Leonardo da Vinci, the "ideal" Western or Caucasian face can be divided into three equal horizontal sections by drawing lines through the forehead, the eyebrows, the base of the nose, and at the lower end of the chin. Additionally, the face can be divided into five vertical segments, each the width of one eye. If a part of the face is "out of proportion" to the other facial features, correction can often provide much better facial harmony. From the side or profile view, the projection of the chin should be in line or just behind the lower lip. Deficiencies may be improved with a chin augmentation which becomes more apparent when evaluating for a rhinoplasty or nose altering surgery.

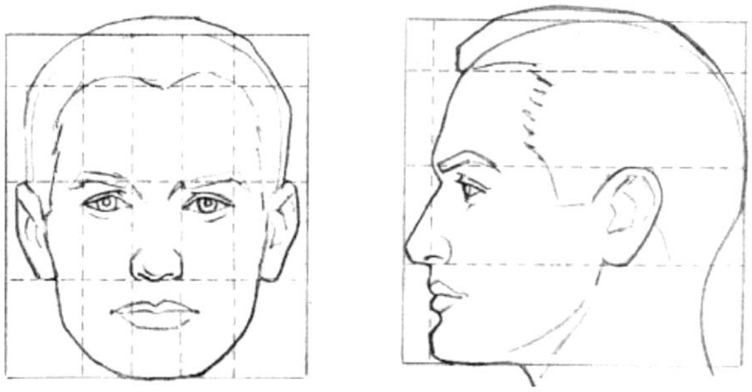

Leonardo da Vinci's "ideal" facial proportions are demonstrated by these diagrams.

## The Consultation: Conferring with Dr. Guy

The first step towards evaluating your rejuvenation options is to schedule a consultation. This is accomplished by either calling our office (832-956-1040) or contacting us on line via our website (www.DrGuyFacialPlastics.com/Contact) after which one of the members of our staff will contact you within 1 business day. Patients who have time schedules to meet (getting back to work, school, conferences, etc.) or who wish to have the surgery as soon as possible, should let us know at the time of scheduling the consultation. This way we can reserve a period in our surgery schedule, but no spot is guaranteed until payment has been received.

On your consultation day, you will have had the chance to fill out your paperwork online through our secure patient portal at your convenience prior to the visit or in the office on the day of your consultation, whichever is more suitable for you.

Upon your arrival, you will be promptly greeted by a member of our excellent staff who will be there to assist you.

Once the paperwork is complete, a series of photographs will be taken to provide useful planning material as well as to help evaluate your results after treatment.

During the consultation visit we will discuss your desires, examine the condition(s) you wish to have addressed, and I will provide you an expert opinion regarding what can be accomplished. A complete review of your medical history will be obtained to verify you are healthy enough to undergo the planned treatments. In some instances, additional testing may be required. This can include laboratory work, electrocardiogram, or consultation with other medical specialists. It is also important to realize that many patients will require a letter of medical clearance from their primary care physicians to verify that they are healthy enough for surgery and that needed health information has not inadvertently been omitted.

At the conclusion of your consultation, I may prescribe medications and will provide you with additional instructions in preparation for the planned treatments.

A thorough and complete consultation takes time. This is your chance to get to know me and the staff and vice versa. This meeting lays the foundation on which our relationship will be built. Choosing to undergo any cosmetic surgery is a deeply personal choice, and a significant amount of time is allotted for this first meeting. Please be prepared to be at the Clinic for a couple of hours.

## Consultation Fees

Special knowledge and skill are necessary to reach an expert opinion on whether or not a cosmetic operation is possible or even indicated for you. The consultation should provide you with a great deal of information about your particular problem, even if surgery is not recommended.

You must realize that even though surgery may not be recommended for you, it requires preparation time, skill, judgement, and experience on my part to arrive at this conclusion. You are purchasing the time and advice of a surgeon, similar to what is done with an accountant or attorney. Payment for consultation is due on the day of service. Of course, any consultation fees paid will be directed towards the costs of any procedures or treatments performed.

## Scheduling Your Surgery

Following your consultation, if it is mutually agreed that surgery is the recommended treatment, a time on the surgical schedule will be reserved for you. It is helpful for you to have some idea about your future plans prior to coming to the consultation, and we encourage you to bring your calendar. As mentioned above, if your schedule is restrict-tive or you would like to have surgery as-soon-as-possible, please indicate this at the time you schedule your consultation so a time on the surgical schedule can be tentatively reserved. Unavoidably, schedules can change, yours and ours, but please notify us immediately if a problem arises which might necessitate rescheduling. We pledge to do likewise.

## The Costs of Surgery

We realize that for most people, cost is a major factor in deciding to have plastic surgery. A number of factors are involved in the total cost for treatment:

1. As all patients have an individualized plan created, some cases are more complicated than others
2. The operating room costs and any overnight stay fees or fees for cosmetic surgery are borne by the patient. Fees with local area facilities have been negotiated to help lower the costs.
3. My skill in the operating room allows for improved efficiency which decreases the time in the operating room. This helps to both lower your costs and lower the risks of any anesthetics required in the operating room.

Throughout the world, prepayment is customary for cosmetic plastic surgery. A patient seeking an elective plastic surgical operation desires an improvement in appearance. Since this does not constitute an emergency, the patient should have sufficient time to plan ahead and arrange his or her finances. It is our policy that a $1,000 non-refundable deposit be paid as a down payment in order to secure your position on the surgical schedule with the remaining balance paid fourteen (14) days prior to the date of surgery. Cancellations made less than fourteen (14) days prior to surgery are subject to a $500 cancellation fee. This policy serves to assure the surgeon that the patient is not undertaking elective surgery which he or she may be unable to afford. There are also financing options including Care Credit which we accept.

Those portions of your surgery which are considered "functional" or "medically necessary" may be covered under your insurance plan. We will be happy to submit the paperwork on your behalf to your insurance, but we can make no guaranty regarding the likelihood that the insurance company will pay. For procedures which are deemed to have both a cosmetic and functional component, the patient will be responsible for all of the costs deemed to be strictly "cosmetic." It is not possible to fill out insurance forms so that it appears the work done was not for cosmetic purposes. This is both ethically wrong and illegal. We appreciate your understanding of this policy.

## Operating Room and Facility Fees

With each cosmetic procedure performed the patient is responsible for the operating room, facility fees, and other related costs. These charges are separate and apart from the surgeon's fee. Facilities are available in the clinic for minor procedures, but for procedures requiring intravenous sedation, this will be performed elsewhere for your safety. We have negotiated with local facilities to provide for improved fees, but beyond that, we have no control over their charges. The fees are usually based on an hourly basis for operating room time. As Dr. Guy is skilled and efficient in the operating room, this does help to lower your costs. You will have access to the proposed fees prior to scheduling any surgery so there will be no surprises. You should know your entire expected bill for cosmetic surgery before leaving on your day of consultation.

Because of variances in insurance companies, the amount to be paid by the patient cannot be exactly determined ahead of time for non-cosmetic procedures, but an estimate can be provided. Please ask if you have any questions and before you consent to becoming a patient at our facility.

## Laboratory and Medical Work Up

Prior to having surgery, for many patients we require a letter of "medical clearance" from your doctor. If you do not have a regular doctor, we can help to arrange an evaluation with a primary care physician in the area. In addition, it is sometimes necessary to perform laboratory tests, electrocardiograms, and chest x rays depending on your age and health. These are routinely performed for your safety based on established national guidelines.

## Developing a Long-Term Doctor-Patient Relationship

The sections of this chapter have dealt a lot with the "business" side of the medical treatment. The reason is because cosmetic medicine is different from other aspects of medicine in that the patient bears the expense of treatment. It is because of this that it is so important that patients understand exactly what they are purchasing. It is for this reason that the above policies have been developed as following them helps to lead to a long-term relationship between us.

During your consultation, it is necessary for us to get to know all your thoughts concerning the surgery you are requesting. As a team, we will do our best to inform you about your surgery, pre and post-operative care, explain what to expect along the way, and answer any questions you may have. The answers to most of your questions should be found in this book, but please feel free to ask any questions you have about your proposed surgery or our policies. It is better to ask questions than to take anything for granted, and we are here to help you.

An important concept to keep in mind is that healing takes time. Following plastic surgery, we will ask you to return at set intervals for us to monitor how well you are healing. <u>Keeping these appointments and following instructions are essential for you to obtain the best possible result in the most expedient manner.</u>

# Chapter 3

## Surgical Protocol and Post-Operative Care

**Where Can Surgery Be Performed?**

**The Day of Surgery**

**After Your Surgery: Responsible Recovery and Follow-Up**

**Patient Post-Operative Reminders**

**A Closing Thought**

## Where Can Surgery Be Performed?

There are many available locations for surgery to be performed. May of our procedures, including facelifts, can be performed in our Clinic on the right patients. The benefit to this is the cost savings available to you when compared to other locations.

For procedures requiring a greater degree of sedation or for those who are more nervous, these can be performed in either the hospital or local surgical centers. The nature of the surgery and your overall health will help to determine which location is the best for you. For most cosmetic procedures for overall healthy patients these will take place at one of the local surgical centers as this offers cost savings to you. The hospital is always an option if you request a cosmetic procedure to be performed there pending operating room availability. Usually, this location is reserved for patients with other medical problems who would benefit from having more resources available.

For reconstructive cases covered by insurance, your insurance company often dictates where the procedure will occur based on existing contracts with facilities. It is not always possible to operate only where your insurance company dictates as I will not have privileges at every possible location. We will attempt to inform you of this prior to your procedure to prevent any surprises with expenses, but from a logistic standpoint with insurance companies this is not always possible, nor feasible in the case of more urgent reconstruction

## The Day of Surgery

I like to say that your surgery day really begins the day before surgery. It is best to get all of your busy work taken care of so you can be ready to relax and be pampered for your recovery period. Since you cannot eat or drink anything after midnight the night before surgery, I recommend you have a meal later in the evening (around 8 or 9 pm) and eat a meal heavier in protein. This will help you stay full for a longer period of time. As a good night sleep is always nice, I will prescribe you a prescription sleeping pill so you can wake up feeling refreshed and ready for your surgery. Although it is not required to take this sleeping aid, most patients will feel better the next morning if they did take it.

On the day of surgery, the exact protocol depends on where your surgery is taking place. Wherever it is, you will be called by the surgical center prior to the day of surgery with special instructions on when and where to meet. You will still have a chance to see me prior to being given any medications that will relax you. Once I see you and go over the operative plan, I will make several marks on your face to again verify we have planned for you what you expect. Once that takes place, your anesthetist will provide you with further medications to make you sleepy and more relaxed before going to the operating room.

The operating room is meant to be a very pleasant and pain free experience. Depending on your surgery, you will be given either a twilight anesthetic (similar to a colonoscopy) and local anesthesia but you retain no recollection of the procedure, or a general anesthetic will be used. The plan can be discussed with the anesthesia team but in the end the anesthetist has the final say on what he or she feels is in your best interest. Regardless of the type of anesthesia used, you should rest assured it will be a pleasant experience for you. We purposely choose a plan that will help keep you as comfortable and relaxed as possible before, during, and after the operation so try not to be apprehensive. Most patients will say the experience was much better and easier than they thought it would be.

When you awake from surgery, you may or may not have a dressing in place. Please refer to the other portions of this book that correspond to the surgery you are having for more specific instructions.

## After Your Surgery: Responsible Recovery and Follow-Up

Upon discharge from your location of surgery, if you are staying with our sitter you or a responsible adult will have brought the medications which were prescribed pre-operatively. Otherwise, a responsible adult will be able to take you home. In addition to what is provided in this book, you will be provided instructions for post-operative care based on the procedures you underwent. You will also be given a follow up appointment in the Clinic. The follow-up appointment is usually the day after discharge.

After your surgery it will be necessary to monitor your healing during regular clinic hours. This is usually the first day after surgery, possibly again during the first week, then at one week, two weeks, one month, three months, six months, and one year. There is never any charge for any cosmetic post-operative visits. These are merely designed to make sure you are healing in the best way possible. The actual timing of your follow-up will vary based on the surgery you underwent. For some procedures, it may take an entire year for your healing to be "complete," so we do urge you to keep your postoperative appointments. If a problem were to arise, we will have follow-up more frequently until the issue has passed.

## Patient Post-Operative Reminders

1. Don't try to evaluate the results of surgery too soon. In the beginning we are only evaluating the healing.
2. Healing times vary from one person to another, so don't try to compare your healing process to another's.
3. Swelling and bruising go away with time.
4. Scars tend to improve with time.
5. Thick scars may be improved with steroid injections.
6. Tightness indicates swelling. Don't pull against it as it can lead to poor healing and affect your cosmetic result.
7. Tissues that begin to sag after surgery are a result of continued aging.
8. Loose skin that develops after surgery was not left behind. It is the result of continued aging.
9. Follow all instructions.
10. Please DO NOT ASK FOR PERMISSION TO BREAK THE RULES. They have been created to help you get the best result.

## A Closing Thought

It is important to realize that although the information provided here should be quite helpful to aid in your understanding my approach and philosophy to plastic surgery, this is only a general protocol. Variations and exceptions to the information do exist. All patients should read the chapter on scar revision on page 115 as it provides very useful information regarding the healing process following surgery. Specific postoperative instructions for each procedure can be found at the end of each respective surgical section. I would recommend you read this prior to your consultation for the procedures you are interested in undergoing.

# Chapter 4

## Surgery of the Nose

**Why rhinoplasty?**
**When is the best age for surgery?**
**The Plan**
**The Surgical Protocol**
**The "Ideal" Nose**
**Nasal Breathing Problems**
**Nasal Fractures: Old and New**
**After Nasal Surgery**
**Points To Remember About Rhinoplasty**
**Post-Operative Information:**
*Swelling*
*Discoloration*
*Hemorrhage*
*Pain*
*Insomnia*
*Depression*
*Keep A Stiff Upper Lip*
*Nasal Blockage and Decongestants*
*Cleaning the Nose*
*Resuming Activities*
*Dryness of the Lips*
*Temperature*
*Medications*
*Weakness*
*Bathing and Hair Care*
*Your First Post-Op Clinic Visit*
*Returning to Work or School*
*Injury to the Nose*
*Quick Check Post-Operative Instructions*
*Remember the things you were told before your operation, namely*
*Report to the Clinic Any*

# Why Rhinoplasty?

Rhinoplasty is the term used for surgery on the outside of the nose. This is commonly performed with surgeries of the septum (the midline structure inside the nose) and called a septorhinoplasty. This includes surgeries designed to improve both breathing (function) and appearance (form). The operation can be quite complex removing excess bone and cartilage while reshaping or rearranging the existing tissue. In some cases, it involves building up the nose which may require cartilage from other areas.

Most rhinoplasties are performed to help improve the appearance, function, or both. This may simply mean bringing the nose into harmony with the rest of the face (see facial analysis on page 20). As children, most noses are very cute and "button-like." Around puberty the nose begins to grow along with the rest of the face. This is very often when humps begin to appear, especially if one's parent also had a hump. As one ages, the nose can become progress-sively enlarged with development of a more noticeable hump and dropping of the nasal tip which can even affect breathing. And of course, any trauma to the nose can certainly affect both the appearance and breathing.

Like faces, every nose is different. Some noses are too long, some too wide, some have large humps, some project away from the face too much and others not enough, and so on. Since rhinoplasty is as much artistic in nature as it is scientific, rarely are any two noses identical. It is because of this that we strive to make each patient's nose fit his or her face instead of giving everyone the same nose.

Many factors go into deciding the best way to approach a nose. This includes your height, age, how thick your skin is, ethnicity, desire to keep any ethnically identifying traits, and other features related to your face. I strive to achieve a natural looking nose rather than one that gives the appearance of an "operated" nose. The ways to accomplish this will be discussed at your consultation.

# When is the best age for surgery?

There are two aspects to consider when contemplating surgery. The first is whether there is an impairment of breathing, and the second is whether the nose is affecting your self-esteem. In children, the nose grows around the age of puberty. There are a few special areas in the nose that help it grow appropriately. Once a child is mature then surgery can be considered for cosmetic purposes. There is no set age but in females it is around a year after the development of menarche (menstruation). In males it tends to be a little bit older but once they quit growing in height it is a good time. Early correction of unwanted nasal deformities can often give young people more self-confidence which can improve self-esteem, interaction with others, and school performance. It is imperative that anyone under age 18 be accompanied by a parent at the time of consultation.

On the other end of the spectrum there are a good number of patients presenting over age 40 for primary rhinoplasty. These patients may have always disliked their noses and finally have the means to address it. In other situations, a nose they had learned to live and breathe through is no longer functioning as well causing nasal obstruction. In other words, it is never too late to undergo a rhinoplasty.

## The Plan

Prior to surgery your photographs will be taken. Through the use of 3-dimensional computer software, a general idea of what may be accomplished will be provided, although no guarantees are made based on the software generated photo. It is merely a tool to help us agree upon a realistic goal to help guide the surgical planning. The operation is then planned to not only improve the shape of the nose but also to improve its harmony with the rest of the face.

## The Surgical Protocol

Following most rhinoplasties, you will notice there is a splint on the outside of your nose. This helps to serve two functions. It limits the amount of swelling that takes place and it also helps to keep structures where I want them to heal. This is especially important if controlled incisions in the bones were required to help improve the shape of the nose. This is in contrast to the "breaking" of the nose that was performed in the past. This external splint generally stays in place for 7 days. No packing is placed on the inside of the nose in the traditional sense. Packing leads to a very uncomfortable healing period and is not usually required except in extreme cases. It also tends to cause more swelling and bruising which is another reason packing is avoided. If work is performed on the septum, then splints made of two small pieces of Silastic (a silicone like plastic) may be placed on the inside of the nose. Small pieces of an absorbable material may also be placed inside to help the healing process. A drip dressing may be present the first night which helps protect your clothes. Most patients are able to go home or a local area hotel the same day as surgery.

## The "Ideal" Nose

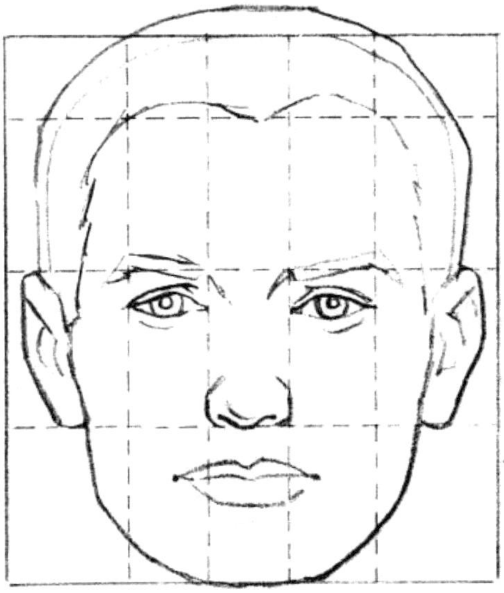

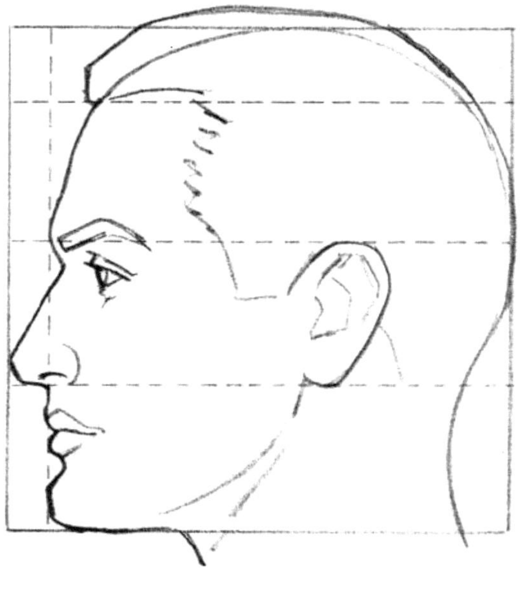

The "ideal" facial proportions based on Western societal norms are demonstrated in this illustration. The nose should fit into the middle one-third of the face as depicted here. From a profile view, the chin should be in line with the lower lip or in females just behind this line.

## Nasal Breathing Problems

One of the more common causes of breathing difficulties is a "deviated" or crooked nasal septum. The septum is a bony and cartilaginous partition that divides the inside of the nose into two sides. If it is dislocated or leans to one side it can interfere with the flow of air through one or both sides of the nose. The nose will naturally cycle with breathing from one side to the other. This helps to prevent the nasal mucosa from drying out. This cycle can last from an hour to several hours. This may be the reason some people notice their nose is intermittently congested but that they never breathe out of one side. We will evaluate the inside of the nose and attempt to improve the airway if we feel it might be improved with corrective surgery.

Even though surgery can often straighten the mechanical obstruction in a crooked nose to improve breathing, the membranes lining the inside of the nose can become swollen from one or more of the following conditions:

- Allergies (hay fever)
- Changes in temperature or environmental factors
- Viral infections (colds)
- Bacterial infections such as sinusitis
- Emotional disturbances, especially crying
- Over-use of over-the-counter nasal decongestant sprays such as Afrin or 12-hour nasal sprays
- Pregnancy and oral contraceptive pills
- Irritants in the air such as cigarette smoking or potpourri
- Certain common medications for blood pressure such as beta blockers

Conditions that cause swelling of the membranes are not corrected by surgery. However, if the patient has a deviated septum and membrane conditions, then correction of the septum frequently makes it easier for the patient to tolerate the membrane swelling. I can also recommend treatments to improve these membrane conditions if needed. At certain times, I may recommend you see an allergist if you are no longer responding to the first line treatments.

## Nasal Fractures: Old and New

The nose is the most commonly injured structure on the face. This is because of its prominence and central location. The bones are also quite weak. When the nose has been injured, fractures and/or dislocations of the nasal bones or cartilages may occur. This leads to a significant amount of swelling. As long as this swelling is present, it is often difficult to diagnose these breaks. Standard X-rays are of limited value since the cartilage, which is easily fractured, cannot be seen with them. CT scans may confirm breaks but they are often not necessary unless there is concern for other injuries. The biggest factors in determining if a fracture is present is 1) does the nose look different or crooked and 2) was there any bleeding that occurred from the inside of the nose. If either of these are present then the likelihood of a break is very high.

As the swelling subsides, the nose may appear more crooked or deformed which was masked by the swelling. Furthermore, airway obstruction which was thought a result of swelling may persist as the breaks in the nose obstruct air flow. Although nasal fractures are not true emergencies, they usually should be repaired within four weeks with the sooner the better. Patients who feel they have broken their nose should be seen the same day as there is a rare but devastating complication which, if not evaluated promptly, can lead to serious cosmetic and functional problems with collapse of the nose. Fractures seen within the first day can, in a select group of patients, be corrected in the clinic. For most patients, correction will require a trip to the operating room. I will make specific recommendations in each individual case depending upon the existing circumstances.

*In some cases, desired changes in the size or shape of the external appearance of the nose can be made while correcting the fractures. These will fall under cosmetic improvements which your insurance will not cover unless directly related to your recent injury.* If you wish to have such alterations considered, let us know when you make your appointment. It would be both unethical and illegal for me to indicate that these cosmetic changes are functional in nature in order to have your insurance cover them.

## After Nasal Surgery

It is important for the first 48 hours to take it easy to minimize the risk of bleeding. For the first 24 hours stay in a recliner and only get up to go to the bathroom. For the next 24 hours it is acceptable to walk around the house, but continue to take it easy and use the recliner for both relaxation and sleeping. After the first 48 hours, the patient is urged to remain out of bed and elevated while sleeping at home. Being in an upright position will decrease swelling and accelerate healing. Avoid any activity that increases blood flow to the nose to prevent a nose bleed. This means keeping your head above your heart, avoid straining, avoid the heat, and avoid exercise. You will usually be prescribed an antibiotic to be taken regularly and pain medication to be taken as needed. It is important to avoid any over the counter pain medications other than Tylenol (acetaminophen) during this period to prevent nasal bleeding. It is also important to only take medications as directed by us to avoid taking too much Tylenol. Salt water nasal sprays are also used to help keep the nose moist and more comfortable. The bottle should never be placed into the nose. Rather, you will lay down on the bed and drip the salt water into your nose. Placing the bottle into the nose could cause damage and affect the result of surgery.

You will be seen during the first week to help clear out any debris or crusting that is developing in the nose. This allows you to breathe more easily. The protective splint and dressings on the nose are removed in the Clinic about one week following surgery. Most patients are able to return to work or school that same day, but continue to avoid any activities that increase the heart rate or blood flow to the face. During this time, he/she must be very careful that the nose is not injured in any way and that it is protected from prolonged exposure to direct sunlight. Regular sun exposure is acceptable. Eye glasses must not be worn unless they are supported from the forehead or cheeks or resting on the external splint.

At the end of the first week when the nasal dressings are removed some swelling of the nose (which the patient feels more than he/she or anyone else sees) is present but progressively diminishes over the next several weeks. This swelling also causes the nose to have a turned-up appearance so do not be alarmed. Generally speaking, about 80% of the swelling disappears by two (2) weeks and 90% by two (2) months. The remainder disappears at the rate of about 1% per month. The "final" result is not present for about one year, occasionally longer. It is very important to be patient, especially at the beginning when we are only evaluating healing, not the results.

When patients have associated breathing problems requiring work to be done on the nasal septum (the internal partition in the middle of the nose), there may be varying amounts of nasal blockage for several weeks after surgery. This can be improved with more frequent clinic visits where I remove obstructing material. If this is not sufficient, topical decongestants may be used for a short period if approved. Other topical medications may also be used if cleared by Dr. Guy such as nasal steroids which help to decrease inflammation. Just as with the salt water sprays, the bottle should not be placed inside the nose to avoid damaging the surgical work.

## Points to Remember About Rhinoplasty

1. There is as much swelling on the inside of the nose as the outside. The nose will be turned up when the bandages come off. Patients should not expect to see the final result at that time. Swelling can be minimized by following the post-operative instructions.
2. With thicker skin, it takes longer for the nose to assume its final shape. Thicker skin, like a sponge, holds on to the swelling a little longer. Each case is different and in my preoperative evaluation, I will attempt to explain the skin limitations in your situation. To help the swelling, patients with thick skin should anticipate receiving steroid injections to the nose monthly after the surgery. This is almost to be expected to help attain the best result.
3. Most of the work is done from the inside of the nose, often aided by the use of a small incision in the skin between the nostrils. A second incision may be necessary to make flaring or wide nostrils smaller. In this case, an incision can be made in the crease where the side of the nostril adjoins the upper lip and cheek. Because this is located in a natural body fold, the scar is practically invisible within a few weeks. With time these incisions become inconspicuous.
4. Patients should remember that in any nose surgery there is a limit to the corrective procedures possible or recommended. The surgical goal is improvement in the existing conditions, not to match the ideal which might be present in one's mind. Some of the limiting factors in rhinoplasty are:
    a. The existing size and shape of the nose
    b. The contour and shape of the face

c. The texture and thickness of the skin
d. The inclination of the chin, lip, and forehead
e. The depth of the angle between the forehead and the nose
f. The height of the individual
g. The healing powers of your tissues
h. Facial asymmetry

5. It is frequently necessary to correct a receding or protruding chin at the time of nose surgery to provide harmony of the facial features. (See section on Chin Augmentation-Mentoplasty)
6. Noses that have been severely injured (as from athletic injuries, or an accident), those which are markedly crooked, or those which have had a previous operation which left the patient with an unsatisfactory result are technically more difficult to correct. This means about 10% of the time another operation is required to get the final result. This also means the vast majority are corrected with a single surgery.
7. Analyze your face and nose from the front and the side in your mirror at home and study how it relates to your other facial features. Look to see if one nostril is different or if your nose is crooked. Most faces have several asymmetries because the face develops from two sides which merge during development. Some of these asymmetries are not correctable with surgery but some are. During your consultation we will discuss your desired alterations and explain our recommendations to you with the aid of computer imaging software.

# Post-Operative Information

The following are designed to answer practically every question that may arise following rhinoplasty. You and your family should read the instructions several times to familiarize yourselves thoroughly with them. Attempt to follow them faithfully, because those who do so generally have the smoothest postoperative course. This, of course, favors proper healing and a better result.

### Swelling

Every operation, no matter how minor, is accompanied by swelling of the surrounding tissues. The swelling is due to the new tissue fluids brought into the area by the body to promote healing. The increased blood supply to the region is responsible for the pink color of the skin and in some of the "discoloration" associated with surgery. When these healing fluids are no longer required, the tissues release them and they are absorbed through the bloodstream.

The amount of swelling varies from person to person, but it seems to occur more in the face because the looseness of the tissues makes the features appear distorted. It is usually greater when both the inside (septum) and outside of the nose have been operated upon than when surgery is done on the inside (septum) only. You may be given medicine before the operation to attempt to keep swelling at a minimum.

You must be willing to accept temporary swelling and discoloration which occurs following such operations. Though usually visually disconcerting, most people feel it is a small inconvenience to pay for the physical and psychological improvement they experience.

The swelling will tend to increase for the first few days after surgery, reaching its peak on the third day. It may also become more pronounced along the jaw line and is generally worse when you first rise in the morning (proof that it is better to stay upright as much as possible during the day!). This is not serious and is not an indication that something is going wrong with your healing.

The main thing to remember is that swelling eventually subsides.

You can help the swelling to subside in several ways:

1. Stay upright (sitting, standing, walking around) as much as possible beginning the second day after your surgery. Of course, you should rest when you are tired, preferably in a recliner to remain upright.
2. Avoid bending over or lifting heavy things for two (2) weeks. Besides increasing the swelling, this may raise the blood pressure and cause bleeding from your nose.
3. Avoid hitting or bumping your nose. Along this line it is wise not to pick up small children who often have unpredictable movements, and you should sleep alone for two (2) weeks after your operation to avoid being bumped by your significant other.
4. Sleep in a recliner at 30 to 40 degrees to improve the swelling. Try not to roll over on your nose although once you fall asleep you will have little control over this.
5. We recommend you use ice compresses consisting of a moistened cold wash towel (not an ice bag) applied in an inverted "V" across the top of the nose and covering each eye as much as possible during the first three (3) days after surgery. Beyond this probably will not help, but if it feels good, you can continue to use them. Avoid getting your nasal splint wet so make sure the towels have been wrung out.
6. Avoid sunning the face for prolonged periods for one (1) month after surgery. Casual sun exposure occurring during your normal daily activities are not harmful.
7. Do not tweeze the eyebrows for (1) week.
8. When bathing, avoid getting the nasal dressing wet; if it becomes loose, let us know.
9. Avoid "sniffing" or constantly, forcibly trying to pull air through the nose as some people do when their noses feel blocked. This will not relieve the sensation of blockage—it will only aggravate it because the suction created on the inside will cause more swelling and may produce bleeding.
10. Avoid constantly rubbing the nostrils and base of the nose with Kleenex or a handkerchief. Not only will this aggravate the swelling, but it could also cause an infection, bleeding, or the accumulation of excessive scar tissue inside the nose. Use a drip dressing instead if the discharge is excessive.
11. Report any excessive bleeding that persists after applying cold compresses and pressure, using a nasal decongestant spray, and lying down (head elevated) for 15 minutes. If there is brisk bleeding or you are concerned, please notify our office (832-956-1040).

**Discoloration**

Following surgery, it is not unusual to have varying amounts of discoloration around the face, usually under the eyes or around the corners of the mouth. Like swelling, the discoloration may become more pronounced for one (1) or two (2) days after you have been discharged; it usually does not last for more than a week, all the while decreasing in intensity. The measures that help the swelling subside will also help the discoloration. You can camouflage the discoloration, to some extent, by using makeup.

### Hemorrhage

Whenever the nasal passages are blocked (as when you have a cold or allergy), the nasal glands produce more mucous than normal. Your nose is blocked from the swelling resulting from your operation, so you can expect more mucous drainage for several days. It will be blood-tinged and should cause you no concern unless the drainage becomes frankly bloody and flows profusely as when one cuts a finger.

If hemorrhage does occur, use a nasal decongestant spray, elevate the head, apply ice compresses about the nose, neck and face, and report it by telephone to 832-956-1040 immediately for further instructions.

Avoid bending over and lifting heavy objects, hitting your nose, and removing any blood clots, etc., from within the nostrils.

### Pain

There is usually little pain following rhinoplasty, but the individual may experience a bruised sensation as a result of postoperative swelling. As is usually the case with such things, this seems worse at night and when one becomes nervous. Unfortunately, the commonly prescribed drugs which relieve pain often cause sensations of light-headedness, especially in the immediate post-operative period making recovery more cumbersome. Therefore, I recommend trying the application of cold compresses and Tylenol as prescribed before resorting to narcotic based drugs.

If the above are not effective, you may take one of the pain relievers prescribed as instructed, but do not mix it with alcohol or operate any heavy machinery while taking pain medication.

### Insomnia

A sleeping aid is routinely prescribed for all patients. This helps patients get a good night sleep before surgery as well as afterwards. These should be used as prescribed at night time only. They should never be mixed with alcohol and you should not drive while using these medications.

Both pain medications and sleeping pills may produce a "hangover" when they wear off and contribute to depression and fatigue. Therefore, they should only be used as needed.

### Depression

It is not unusual for an individual to go through a period of "the blues" for a few days after surgery because, no matter how much he/she wanted the operation beforehand and how much they were told about what to expect postoperatively, they are disturbed when they see swelling and/or discoloration about their face.

Be realistic and realize that this sensation will subside shortly. The best "treatment" consists of keeping busy with the details of post-operative care and trying to divert one's mind to other activities such as reading or watching television.

### Keep a Stiff Upper Lip

The upper lip is a key area in rhinoplasty surgery since work is frequently done in this area. Therefore, you should not move it excessively as long as the bandage is in place so that the healing tissues are not disturbed.

Toward this end:

1. Avoid excessive grinning and smiling.
2. Don't pull the upper lip down such as when applying lip-stick or Chap-stick.
3. The upper teeth should be cleansed with toothpaste on a face cloth for the first week to avoid accidentally hitting the area below the nose. The lower teeth should be brushed as usual with a toothbrush.
4. Avoid chewing gum or foods that are hard to chew. Soups, mashed potatoes, stewed chicken, hamburger steak, or any easily chewable foods are recommended.
5. You may decide to continue wearing a drip-dressing because of mucous drainage after you leave the Clinic or hospital. If the dressing becomes "stuck" it may be loosened with a few drops of hydrogen peroxide.

### Nasal Blockage and Decongestants

Nasal blockage is to be expected after rhinoplasty and will gradually subside over a period of time. There is as much swelling on the inside of the nose as there is on the outside. The first week can feel like having a cold because of the difficulty breathing through your nose. I recommend the use of nasal saline sprays (NOT RINSES) to help keep the nose moist. The bottle, or any bottle, should not be placed inside your nose at any time. If needed, lay down on the bed and drip the solution into your nose. With severe congestion you can also use topical decongestants such as Afrin IF CLEARED BY DR. GUY and never for longer than 3 continuous days to prevent worsening congestion.

### Cleaning the Nose

Don't blow the nose at all for fourteen (14) days. After that you can blow through both sides at once—do not compress one side as this can disrupt the work performed at surgery and it also creates more force with blowing which can damage the work performed on the inside of the nose. This helps to prevent you from dislodging a clot and causing bleeding. This should be continued for a total of four (4) weeks following surgery.

You may clean the outside of the nose and the upper lip with cotton-tipped applicators (Q-tips) moistened with hydrogen peroxide as soon as you return home from the Clinic or hospital, but don't rub vigorously. It is a gentle rolling over of the areas so as not to disrupt any stitches or clots. At times, I may also recommend a topical antibiotic ointment to be applied to the areas to help with healing.

Soon after the bandage has been removed, the outside of the nose should be cleaned with a mild soap on a cotton ball twice daily to remove the oily material that is produced by the skin glands. Failure to do this will lead to prolonged swelling and the development of pimples.

### Resuming Activities

You may sleep without the head of the bed elevated after two (2) weeks but if you can last for 4 weeks, you will notice the swelling go away even faster. For the first two (2) weeks you should wear clothing that fastens either in the front or the back rather than the type that must be pulled over the head to avoid pulling on the nose.

Avoid any activity that increases your heart rate for two (2) weeks. This includes swimming, weight lifting, cardiovascular exercise, or strenuous athletic activity. No sports that can lead to contact with your nose should be undertaken for six (6) weeks. Joggers may walk after two (2) weeks and jog after three (3) weeks. Start slowly and work your way back to your pre-surgery routine. Tennis players may hit ground strokes in three (3) weeks and resume competition after six (6) weeks. Do not play "doubles" for six (6) weeks.

Avoid sneezing until the bandage is removed. If you need to sneeze, make sure you open your mouth to prevent the rapidly escaping air from passing through your nose.

Eye glasses can be worn as long as the protective dressings remain on the nose the first postoperative week. After that, they must be supported from the forehead or cheeks for a period of about six (6) weeks with tape. We'll show you how this is to be done if you must wear them. This is important, because the pressure of the glasses may change the new contour of the nose if not suspended. Contact lens may be inserted the day after surgery.

### Dryness of the Lips

If your lips become dry from breathing through the mouth it is ok to use a form of Chap Stick or lip balm. Be careful to not purse your lips while applying to avoid pulling on the upper lip.

### Temperature

Generally, the body temperature does not rise much above 100 degrees following rhinoplasty. Any elevation is generally due to the fact that the patient becomes mildly dehydrated because he/she does not drink enough fluids.

Patients will often think they have fever because they feel warm, but, in reality do not. To be sure, you should measure your temperature with a thermometer. Report any persistent temperature above 100 degrees as this could be the sign of a developing infection.

### Medications

Following surgery, you should resume taking all of the medications you were taking prior to surgery with the exception of blood thinners. These should be avoided for one week after surgery unless medically directed by your physician or myself.

You will also be given several other prescriptions. These will include a sleeping pill, pain pill, and antibiotic. The antibiotics should be taken daily as prescribed until they run out. The sleeping pill should be taken only as needed at night time and not within 2 hours of taking your pain pill.

You may also be given an antihistamine and/or decongestant. Directions for taking them will be written on the bottles. Do not take the antihistamine unless you are experiencing sneezing or have excessive mucous drainage. Narcotic based pain relievers and certain sleeping medications can also make people drowsy and add to depression. If your pain is not severe, rely on acetaminophen (Tylenol) and cold compresses if possible. If this does not resolve the pain, your prescribed pain reliever may be taken as directed.

### Weakness

After a person has an anesthetic or any type of operation it is not unusual for him or her to feel weak, have a rapid pulse, break out in "cold sweats," or get dizzy. Because of this, make sure every time you get up for the first 48 hours that someone has a hold of you. You never know when the weakness is going to hit.

This gradually clears up in a few

days without medication. Drink juices and water to stay hydrated!

### Bathing and Hair Care

Tub bathing or showering can be resumed as soon as you feel strong enough after the day of surgery. It is probably best to have assistance standing by on the first couple of occasions. If you elect to shower, having someone in the shower for the first 48 hours would be recommended in case you become weak.

Your hair may be washed, with someone's help, the day after surgery. Take care to keep water off of the nasal dressing and do not use hot water, but warm water is acceptable. Lay your head back in a lavatory or sink as long as the dressings are in place. A hand-held blow dryer may be used for drying.

### Your First Post-Op Clinic Visit

Before going home you should talk with the receptionist at the Clinic and make an appointment for a check-up on the morning following surgery and about a week following your surgery. This should be done because special preparations must be made for your visits in advance of your arrival—these are different from the usual Clinic routine. Depending on your degree of nasal obstruction, you will also be seen another time during the first week to help remove some of the crusting that develops

Don't build up a feeling of fear and anxiety about what is going to be done to you during the post-operative visits. If cleaning is needed, a topical anesthetic and decongestant spray is used to help. At one week, the tape and splint will be removed with the help of a special tape-removing solution to ensure that these come off easily. Likewise, any material inside your nose will be softened so that it comes out easily. There should be no stitches to remove from the inside of your nose because the dissolvable type is used. If your nostrils were narrowed, those stitches are also of the dissolvable type. You will probably feel much better after the first Clinic visit when you see your "new nose."

### Returning to Work or School

The average patient is able to return to school the day the bandages are removed, that is, about a week following surgery. If you don't mind being seen with a nasal splint, some patients will return sooner.

When you should return to work depends on the amount of physical activity and public contact your job involves, in addition to the amount of swelling and discoloration you develop. The average patient may return to work by the eighth to tenth postoperative day, some sooner for desk or computed based jobs.

### Injury to the Nose

Many individuals sustain accidental hits on the nose during the early post-operative period. One need not be too concerned unless the blow is hard or if bleeding or considerable swelling ensues. Report the incident at the next Clinic visit or by telephone if you are sufficiently concerned. After about 6 weeks, a hit hard enough to break the nose would have been able to break it had no surgery been performed in the first place.

### Post-Operative Instructions

Please follow these instructions carefully. You should also review the materials in the consultation book relative to your surgery. Your final result will depend upon how well you care for the treated areas.

**WEEK 1**

DO: Sleep on your back with the head of the bed elevated for 2 weeks.

DO: Use saline sprays (not rinses) to help keep your noise moist and help with the crusting.

DO: Apply cold compresses to the eye and nose area 20 minutes out of every waking hour for the first 3 days.

DO: We recommend moistened cold washcloths soaked in ice water, applied in an inverted V across the top of the nose and covering the eyes once the washcloth is ringed out.

DO: Wear a drip pad under your nose as long as you have drainage from the nose. This avoids excessive manipulation of the nose.

DO: Expect swelling to increase by the 3rd day, then it will gradually start to decrease.

DO: Eat soft foods for the first week. Avoid foods that are hot or cold.

DO: Clean only the entrance of the nostrils as needed with hydrogen peroxide on a cotton swab applicator as demonstrated by Dr. Guy.

DO: Clean the sutures in the creases of each nostril 6 times daily with peroxide and apply antibiotic ointment if your nostrils were narrowed.

DO: Wear contacts or glasses the day after surgery, if desired. Your splint will protect the nose.

* * * * *

DO NOT: Clean passed the entrance of your nostrils at all. You might initiate bleeding.

DO NOT: Blow or sniff through your nose for 14 days.

DO NOT: Brush your top teeth for the first week but you may use your finger with toothpaste or a cloth on your finger with toothpaste as an alternative.

DO NOT: Pucker lips or stretch your upper lip for 1 week (keep a "stiff upper lip").

DO NOT: Use ice bags or aqua packs for compresses over the eyes. Using ice directly on the skin can cause serious damage.

DO NOT: Get the splint on your nose wet. To avoid this while showering, try bending your back to the shower.

DO NOT: Bend over at the waist. Instead squat down to pick up light objects, and no heavy lifting at all for 2 weeks.

DO NOT: Bump or hit your nose. Avoid picking up small children or pets. Sleeping alone is recommended for 2 weeks.

**WEEK 2**

DO: Wear makeup on the nose if desired.

DO: Clean your nose gently with a cotton ball and soap if desired.

DO: Sleep on your back, with the head of your bed elevated for at least 1 more week.

DO: Expect to have some swelling. Generally 80% of the swelling will be gone by the end of the 2nd week and 90% by the end of two months. The final 10% can take up to 12-18 months to resolve.

DO: Start eating regular foods.

DO: Start brushing your teeth with a toothbrush.

DO: Apply a small amount of antibiotic ointment or Vaseline inside each nostril with the tip of your small finger. This will help keep any crusting inside the nostrils soft.

You may blow your nose on the 14th postoperative day if needed. Gently do so by keeping both nostrils open and blowing softly.

* * * * *

DO NOT: Clean passed the entrance of your nostrils.
DO NOT: Attempt any heavy exercise for 1 more week, then progress slowly back to your regular exercise program. Listen to your body. Brisk walking is acceptable at this time.
DO NOT: Attempt heavy lifting.
DO NOT: Bump or hit your nose.
DO NOT: Wear glasses or sunglasses directly on bridge of nose for 6 weeks following the removal of the splint. Glasses must be taped to suspend them from the forehead.

**Remember the things you were told before your operation, namely:**

1. When the bandage is first removed, your nose will appear swollen and turned up too much; this is due to swelling over the nose and in the upper lip. The swelling will begin to subside within a week; however, it will take at least one year for the swelling to disappear completely and for your nose to reach its final shape.
2. In most cases, the discoloration will gradually disappear over a period of seven (7) to ten (10) days.
3. With thicker and oilier skin, it takes longer for the swelling to subside, so be patient.
4. Your upper lip may feel stiff for a while and you may feel that it interferes with your smile. This will disappear within a few weeks.
5. The tip of the nose sometimes feels “numb” after rhinoplasty, but this eventually disappears. The same goes for the upper teeth in the middle (your incisors).
6. Patients who have very oily skin may use rubbing alcohol and cotton balls to remove excess oils from the nasal skin for 2-3 days after the dressings have been removed.
7. Noses that are crooked, have sustained injuries, or have had previous surgery are more difficult to correct. Additional improvement may be obtained with a relatively minor procedure later.
8. Failure to follow these instructions faithfully can lead to certain complications which potentially could jeopardize the desired result.
9. Remember, that the surgery was performed for improvements and that perfection is almost never achieved.

**Report To The Clinic Any:**

1. Temperature elevation greater than 100 degrees
2. Sudden swelling or discoloration.
3. Hemorrhage.
4. Discharge from the wound edges or other evidence of infection.
5. Development of any reaction to medications.

If you have any questions call

832-956-1040

# Chapter 5

## Surgery of the Chin

**Chin Augmentation/Mentoplasty**

**Reduction Mentoplasty**

**After Chin Augmentation**

*Submental Approach*
*Intraoral Approach*
*Post-Operative Instructions*
*Remember the things you were told before your operation, namely*
*Report to the Clinic Any*

# Chin Augmentation/Mentoplasty

Mentum is the Greek word for chin; the suffix "plasty" means to shape or mold. When the chin is too small for the face, augmentation can often produce a dramatic improvement in the overall appearance of the face.

Very often it is necessary to recommend surgery for a receding chin either in connection with a nose job (rhinoplasty), a face lift, liposuction, or even as an isolated procedure. This occurs because the facial plastic surgeon does not consider the chin as an isolated structure. Instead, it is seen as an important feature of the face as a whole. This procedure carries a high success rate and frequently adds the "finishing touch" when reconstructing facial harmony.

During your consultation your chin will be analyzed to determine if augmentation should be considered. Generally speaking, if one examines the profile (side view) in a mirror, the chin projection should be even with a vertical line dropped from the lower lip in males or be slightly behind this line in females. Too much recession of the chin, particularly when accompanied by a slanting forehead, will cause the features to taper to a point in the mid-face if only a rhinoplasty (nasal plastic surgery) is done. Actually, we may advise against any surgery for some individuals unless the projection of the chin can be increased in conjunction with rhinoplasty.

Of course, there are people who desire chin augmentation alone for a receding or "weak" chin. Oftentimes these people will have a very specific constellation of facial findings that goes along with the receding chin. This usually includes difficulty breathing from the nose because of large adenoids (tissue you cannot see at the back of the nose) that when swollen completely block the nose causing mouth breathing. The mouth breathing leads to a high arched palate at the top of the mouth which can affect how your teeth come together. A chin implant can improve the aesthetic appearance of these patients.

For those patients with a receding chin who are interested in a face lift, adding a chin augmentation can both improve facial harmony and improve the appearance of the neck greater than a neck lift without the chin augmentation.

The operation can be performed either through the mouth or under the chin. The approach is determined by any other procedures you are considering. When performed within the mouth, an incision just above the crease between the lower lip and gum is made. Absorbable sutures are used and when the scar "matures," generally, it is well-camouflaged. It can also be performed from below the chin. This is frequently done when performed as part of submental liposuction or a neck lift using an incision that is made in these other procedures.

If performed alone, it can be performed in the clinic under local anesthesia for carefully selected patients. When performed as part of another operation it does not add any extra time to the healing process although a dressing is placed on the chin for a week that otherwise wouldn't have been there.

There are several implant options. The option most commonly used and recommended is a soft medical grade silicone implant. All implants help to increase the chin projection by supporting the soft tissue overlying the mandible or jaw bone. This is the same concept as with breast augmentation wherein an implant is placed under the tissue. In the chin operation, the implant is placed on the jaw bone so that the soft tissues (skin, fat and muscles) rest upon the implant instead of the bone. This material has been widely used for an extended period and has an excellent safety profile.

With chin augmentation one must be willing to accept certain risks that may occur with any surgery on other areas of the body, (i.e., infection, rejection, numbness, swelling, asymmetries, discoloration, distortions, scars, etc.). Although the chin area will be sensitive for a few days, postoperative discomfort is usually negligible. There may be some degree of numbness overlying the chin which resolves over about 3 weeks.

Until most of the swelling has subsided, your lower lip and chin area may feel somewhat full and tight. Do not try to evaluate the results of your surgery too soon. It may take several weeks before the majority of swelling and tightness subsides, sometimes longer.

In those patients who have receding chins and an abnormal bite, i.e., the upper and lower do not meet properly, a chin augmentation may not be the best choice. In these cases, orthodontic evaluation should be considered for a more aggressive surgery whereby the entire mandible (jaw bone) may need to be repositioned. Although we do not offer this more aggressive surgery, we will discuss this with you if you have any questions about it.

## Reduction Mentoplasty

Although it is much more common for the chin to be too small, some chins are too large. The excess bone can be removed or repositioned to help provide better harmony and refine the chin to some extent in select patients. Drastic changes are not recommended because this tends to cause a very droopy chin, almost like a witch.

## After Chin Augmentation

The following are designed to answer practically every question that may arise regarding the "do's" and "don'ts" after surgery. You and your family should read the instructions several times to familiarize yourselves thoroughly with them. Attempt to follow them faithfully, because those who do so generally have the smoothest post-operative course. This, of course, favors proper healing and a better result.

If your chin surgery was performed in conjunction with another procedure, you should also follow the instructions pertaining to that procedure.

As is the case with any operation, you can expect swelling in the postoperative period. The swelling is due to the new tissue fluids brought into the area by the body to promote healing. The increased blood supply to the region is responsible for the pink color of the skin and in some of the "discoloration" associated with surgery. When these healing fluids are no longer required, the tissues release them and they are absorbed through the bloodstream. The increased swelling produces a feeling of tightness and pressure in the chin. This is a normal part of healing and should not produce concern.

You must be willing to accept temporary swelling and discoloration which occurs following such operations. Though usually visually disconcerting, most people feel it is a negligible inconvenience to pay for the physical and psychological improvement they experience.

A tape dressing is usually placed over your chin following surgery. Do not attempt to remove the dressing and try not to get it wet. It is usually removed during the one week post-operative visit to the Clinic.

When the dressings are removed and you first see your new chin, it will be swollen and might look as though it has been over-corrected, but be patient. As the swelling subsides, it should assume a more natural appearance.

You may be tempted to feel the implant with your fingers or explore the suture line under the lip with your tongue. We encourage you not to do this as the implant is adapting to its new tissue bed and manipulation may jeopardize the healing. The skin over the implant has been covered with tape for several days and fingertips contain oil and debris that might cause "pimples" to occur.

Gentle washing of your chin is recommended after the dressings have been removed.

You will be provided with an antibiotic which should be taken until it has been completed. Although this is not usually a painful operation, if you do have pain, use Tylenol ® as instructed. If this does not relieve your pain then it is okay to use the prescribed pain medication. Keep in mind, this medicine tends to make people feel drowsy and can make the recovery period more tedious. Therefore, only use it if needed.

### Submental Approach

If the chin implant was placed through the submental (under the chin) approach, an incision was made in a crease below the chin. The sutures used to close the incision are absorbable. Any remaining suture material usually comes off when the tape covering this incision is removed in about one week. If any sutures do remain, they will also be removed at one week.

### Intraoral Approach

If the implant was placed through the intraoral approach, an incision was made inside the mouth just above the crease between the lip and gum. The sutures used to close this incision are absorbable and need not be removed.

### Post-Operative Instructions

DO: Eat soft foods (soups, Jell-O, puddings, potatoes, etc.) for at least five (5) days after surgery. If the incision was made in your mouth, follow a liquid diet for the first three (3) days.

* * * * *

DO NOT: Manipulate sutures or pull your lower lip forward as it may interfere with the healing.

DO NOT: Eat foods such as nuts, popcorn, grits, etc. if your incision was intraoral, that may leave debris in the lower lip crease as it may irritate the healing suture line.

DO NOT: Force your tongue down into the crease to "feel" the sutures or attempt to clean the debris. This maneuver, too, may interfere with healing.

DO NOT: Use a toothbrush on the lower teeth for the first week if an intraoral incision was made. Instead, use toothpaste on your fingers.

DO NOT: Engage in any activities that can injure your chin for at least three (3) weeks including:

- Contact sports

- Diving or skiing
- Holding small children
- Large crowds
- Manipulating the lower lip

**Remember the things you were told before your operation, namely:**

1. There will be a bandage around your chin. Leave it in place until it is removed in the clinic. It is designed to keep your implant in place during the early healing period.
2. If the incision was made through your mouth, you will be on a liquid diet for the first three (3) days. After that, you can begin a soft diet but avoid any gritty food which could get stuck in your incisions. If the incision was outside of your mouth, you can begin a soft diet the first day after surgery. Soft diets should be continued until seven (7) days after surgery. Your diet can then be advanced to a regular diet as tolerated.
3. Avoid excessive grinning or smiling as this can pull on the implant.
4. Avoid any strenuous activity for the first two (2) weeks after surgery. After this you can begin to resume your previous activity, but listen to your body.
5. It is normal to have some numbness in the chin area. Let us know during your Clinic visits if you have any so that we can monitor the progress of your healing more closely. This should improve over the first few weeks.
6. Because of the proximity of the nerve that provides sensation to the jaw, it is also normal to have some discomfort in your lower teeth after surgery. This will improve as the swelling goes down.
7. When your dressing comes off there will be some swelling and the chin will appear over corrected. This will improve.
8. The average patient is able to return to school the day the bandages are removed. This is about a week after surgery. If you don't mind being seen with a chin splint, some patients will return sooner.
9. When you should return to work depends on the amount of physical activity and public contact your job involves, in addition to the amount of swelling and discoloration you develop. The average patient may return to work by the eighth to tenth postoperative day, some sooner for desk or computer-based jobs.
10. If you notice extreme swelling or redness around the implant, notify us immediately. You should report any drainage from the incision sites.
11. Like other plastic surgical operations, it may take 6-12 months for the last five (5) or ten (10) percent of swelling to disappear, so be patient. We will ask you to return for post-operative visits at several intervals during the first year or so. These visits are necessary for us to monitor the progress of your healing, so please notify us if you have a problem.
12. Failure to follow these instructions faithfully can lead to certain complications which potentially could jeopardize the desired result.

**Report to the Clinic Any:**

1. Temperature elevation greater than 100 degrees
2. Sudden swelling or discoloration.
3. Hemorrhage.
4. Discharge from the wound edges or other evidence of infection.
5. Development of any reaction to medications.

If you have any questions call

832-956-1040

# Chapter 6

## Cheek Augmentation

### Cheek Enhancement

### After Cheek Augmentation

*Post-Operative Instructions*
*Remember the things you were told before your operation, namely*
*Report to the Clinic Any*

# Cheek Enhancement

For centuries, high cheekbones have been a common characteristic of faces considered to be "beautiful." The simplest and least invasive method of enhancing the cheeks is with the use of temporary fillers (see chapter 15). Fillers are useful to get an appreciation for what could be accomplished without the downtime of surgery. When a more permanent correction is desired, it can be accomplished by placing medical grade Silastic implants directly on the facial bones.

When patients elect for the more permanent surgical option, the incisions are usually made inside the mouth and under the upper lip. This allows for the avoidance of any scars on the face. These incisions are closed with absorbable sutures which dissolve within about 7 days.

As a specialist in facial plastic surgery, I analyze the face and attempt to select the appropriate implant for each patient and for each cheek as there are many sizes and shapes available. Rarely are the two sides of the face symmetrical prior to surgery, so one can expect some asymmetry to be present after the operation. During your facial analysis prior to your consultation, you may have noticed this. As is the case with any augmentation procedure there are imponderables, risks, and the possibility that the operation might not reach a patient's expectations. It is important to have realistic expectations including the likelihood of persistence of a slight asymmetry between the two sides.

However, cheek augmentations, like chin augmentations, can provide a finishing touch and better balance for patients seeking improved facial harmony. The procedure can be performed in conjunction with many of the other procedures described in this book, or can be done as an isolated procedure. I do not usually recommend a cheek augmentation at the time of a facelift because the lifting of the facial tissues can frequently restore the cheek close to its more youthful appearance. If a cheek augmentation would be required later a more appropriately sized implant could be chosen.

Although the cheek areas are swollen initially and some bruising may occur, the swelling subsides in a few weeks. Initially the cheeks will appear over corrected but this will improve as the swelling dissipates. The final result will not be apparent until this occurs.

Most patients may return to work or resume "normal" activities within a few days after surgery. Patients are urged to avoid injury to the cheek region for 4-6 weeks to prevent dislodging the implant. After that time, it is unlikely that the implant(s) could be disturbed unless a severe blow were to be received.

You will notice the instructions below are very similar to the instructions provided for a chin implant via an intraoral approach because the concepts and surgical approaches behind the surgeries are similar.

# After Cheek Augmentation

The following are designed to answer practically every question that may arise regarding the "dos" and "don'ts" after surgery. You and your family should read the instructions several times to familiarize yourselves thoroughly with them. Attempt to follow them faithfully, because those who do so generally have the smoothest post-operative course. This, of course, favors proper healing and a better result.

If your chin surgery was performed in conjunction with another procedure, you should also follow the instructions for that procedure.

**Post-Operative Instructions**

DO: Follow a liquid diet for the first three (3) days. After that eat soft foods (soups, Jell-O, puddings, potatoes, etc.) for at least seven (7) days after surgery.

* * * * *

DO NOT: Manipulate sutures or pull the upper lip forward as it may interfere with the healing.

DO NOT: Eat foods such as nuts, popcorn, grits, etc., that may leave debris in the upper lip crease as it may irritate the healing suture line.

DO NOT: Force the tongue into the upper crease to "feel" the sutures or attempt to clean the debris. This maneuver, too, may interfere with healing.

DO NOT: Use a toothbrush on the upper teeth for the first week. Instead, use toothpaste on your fingers.

DO NOT: Engage in any activities that can injure the cheeks for at least three (3) weeks including:

- Contact sports
- Diving or skiing
- Holding small children
- Large crowds
- Manipulating the lower lip

If you should notice extreme swelling or redness around the implant, notify us immediately. You should report any drainage from the incision sites. Sometimes numbness of the cheek can follow surgery. Let us know during your Clinic visits if you have any so that we can monitor the progress of your healing more closely.

Like other plastic surgical operations, it may take 6-12 months for the last five (5) or ten (10) percent of swelling to disappear, so be patient. We will ask you to return for postoperative visits at several intervals during the first year or so. These visits are necessary for us to monitor the progress of your healing, so please notify us if you have a problem.

Failure to follow these instructions faithfully can lead to certain complications which potentially could jeopardize the desired result.

**Remember the things you were told before your operation, namely:**

- You will be on a liquid diet for the first three days. After that, you can begin a soft diet but avoid any gritty food which could get stuck in your incisions. Soft diets should be continued until 7 days after surgery. Your diet can then be advanced to a regular diet as tolerated.
- Avoid excessive grinning or smiling as this can pull on the implant.
- Avoid any strenuous activity for the first two (2) weeks after surgery. After this you can begin to initiate your previous activity, but listen to your body.
- It is normal to have some numbness in the cheek area. This should improve over the first few weeks.
- Because of swelling, the cheeks will initially appear overcorrected. This will improve.
- The average patient is able to return to school by post-operative day 7. If you don't mind being seen with swollen cheeks, some patients will return sooner.
- When you should return to work

depends on the amount of physical activity and public contact your job involves, in addition to the amount of swelling and discoloration you develop. The average patient may return to work by the eighth to tenth postoperative day, some sooner for desk or computed based jobs.

**Report To The Clinic Any:**

1. Temperature elevation greater than 100 degrees
2. Sudden swelling or discoloration.
3. Hemorrhage.
4. Discharge from the wound edges or other evidence of infection.
5. Development of any reaction to medications.

If you have any questions call

832-956-1040

# Chapter 7

# Lip Enhancement

## Lifting and Augmentation

## Postoperative Instructions

## After Lip Enhancement

*Post-Operative Instructions*

*Remember the things you were told before your operation, namely*

*Report to the Clinic Any*

# Lifting and Augmentation

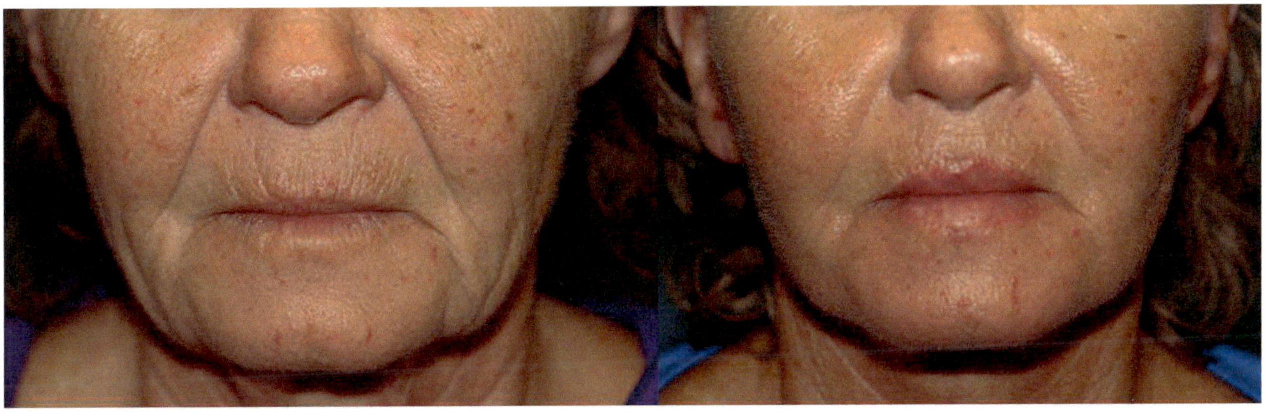

Before After

This patient underwent a lip advancement and lip augmentation with her own collagen. Note the natural appearing full lips 4 months out from surgery. She is wearing no lipstick or lip liner so you can see how well the incisions are camouflaged. It has also improved the fine lines around her mouth even though she has not had any skin resurfacing.

More and more people are becoming interested in having larger, more youthful lips. If you have ever considered lip enhancement but are not sure if it is for you, injectables provide an excellent short-term option. I recommend a hyaluronic acid based filler, such as Juvederm Ultra XC, Restylane Kysse, or RHA Redensity. These tend to last between 6 months and a year. When done properly they can provide a nice natural appearing enhancement with a soft feel. It is important to realize that these are merely temporary and if you like the results, you will need repeat injections. The other option is to consider a longer lasting surgical procedure.

From a surgical standpoint, your lips can also be filled with your own collagen. This is usually harvested at the time of a facelift and the collagen would otherwise be discarded. If you'd like the enhancement, a small tunnel is created on the top and bottom of your lips in which to place the collagen.

The benefit is that it is your own material so you don't have to worry about rejecting the material. It also provides for a natural feel as opposed to some of the permanent implant materials which I do not recommend (such as Gore-Tex or silicone). It is expected that some of your collagen will disappear with time, but the majority of it is retained which is a benefit over temporary fillers.

Another option is the surgical lip lift. There are several options for this. One is performed by removing a strip of the white skin around the lip and advancing the pink skin into the area. This creates more of a full lip by showing more of the pink part of the lip. The scar is placed in a natural junction of the mouth and usually heals quite well as can be seen in the photo above. It is important to realize that lipstick or lip liner may be needed to completely hide this scar. The other options it the "bull horn" lip lift named because the shape of the excision mirrors the shape of the horns of a bull. This involves making an incision just below the nose to elevate the lip. The benefit of this over the direct approach above is the incision is hidden in the shadow of the nose. With either surgical option they tends to make the lip feel a little firmer during the healing process which can last up to a year. However, since this method does not rely on any implanted material such as hyaluronic acid or your own collagen, the gains achieved with the lift are not lost since there is no filler to disappear with time.

For patients over the age of 40, surgery is often combined with a resurfacing procedure such as laser resurfacing, a chemical peel, or dermabrasion for the best results. The resurfacing helps mainly with the wrinkles around the mouth, commonly called "Smoker's lines" although many nonsmokers develop them.

Surgical incisions are either closed with absorbable sutures which usually dissolve within 5-7 days or permanent blue sutures that are removed around day 2 or 3 following the surgery. The incision lines go through the usual maturation process in which the scar is pink and lumpy for a few weeks and eventually blends into the surrounding tissues as it flattens and turns white. It is important to realize that this takes up to a year to complete. Some patients may desire correction of the upper (or lower lip) only. Most, however choose to have both done. I will provide you with my recommendation based on your thorough facial evaluation at the time of your consultation.

Any of the lip procedures can be performed as isolated procedures or may be combined with most of the other plastic surgical operations discussed in this book. Because the lips have such a great blood supply, which is part of the reason they appear red/pink, expect them to be quite swollen after surgery. For several weeks they will appear "over-corrected." Rest assured that as the swelling goes down in the first month or two, they will appear appropriately corrected and enhanced.

## After Lip Enhancement

The following are designed to answer practically every question that may arise regarding the "dos" and "don'ts" after surgery. You and your family should read the instructions several times to familiarize yourselves thoroughly with them. Attempt to follow them faithfully, because those who do so generally have the smoothest post-operative course. This, of course, favors proper healing and a better result.

If your lip enhancement surgery was performed in conjunction with another procedure, you should also follow the instructions pertaining to that procedure.

**Post-Operative Instructions**

DO: Clean your incisions with hydrogen peroxide six (6) times daily and then place the antibiotic ointment in a fine line around the incisions.

DO: Eat soft foods which are easily chewed to prevent straining your lips.

* * * * *

DO NOT: Use straws or strain your mouth with smiling or puckering your lips.

DO NOT: Manipulate sutures or pull your lips forward as it may interfere with the healing.

DO NOT: Apply lipstick or lip liner for the first two weeks

DO NOT: Use your tongue to push on your lips or feel your sutures

**Remember the things you were told before your operation, namely:**

1. You will be on a soft diet for the first week. Your diet can then be advanced to a regular diet as tolerated.
2. Avoid excessive grinning or smiling as this can pull on the incisions.
3. Avoid any strenuous activity for the first two (2) weeks after surgery. After this you can begin to initiate your previous activity, but listen to your body.
4. It is normal to have some numbness in the lips. This should improve over the first few weeks.
5. Because of swelling the lips will initially appear overcorrected. This will improve.
6. When you should return to work depends on the amount of physical activity and public contact your job involves, in addition to the amount of swelling and discoloration you develop. The average patient may return to work by the fifth to tenth postoperative day, some sooner.

**Report to The Clinic Any:**

1. Temperature elevation greater than 100 degrees
2. Sudden swelling or discoloration.
3. Hemorrhage.
4. Discharge from the wound edges or other evidence of infection.
5. Development of any reaction to medications.

If you have any questions call

832-956-1040

# Chapter 8

## Surgery of the Ears

### Otoplasty: Surgery for Prominent and Protruding Ears

### The Surgery

### After Otoplasty

*Postoperative Instructions*
*Remember the things you were told before your operation, namely*
*Report to the Clinic Any*

# Otoplasty: Surgery for Prominent and Protruding Ears

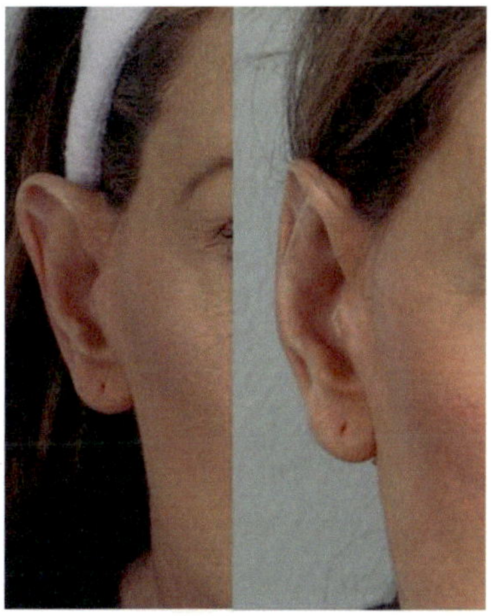

Before After

This patient in her 50s is two months out following bilateral ear pinning surgery. She now feels comfortable wearing a pony tail without having her ears draw attention.

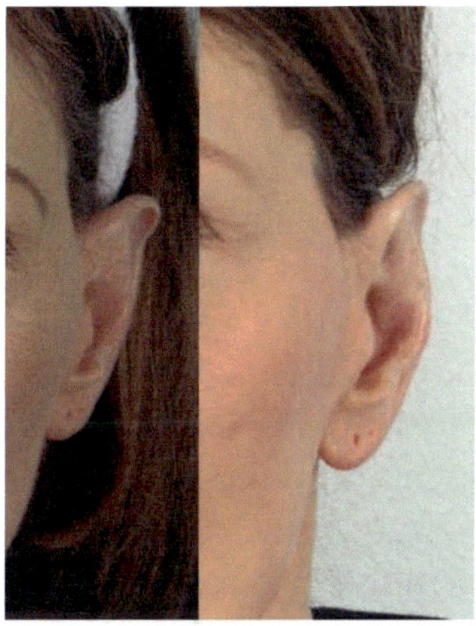

Before After

Otoplasty is the name of the procedure designed to reposition or "pin back" protruding ears. This deformity often causes deeper emotional upset than is generally realized by the patient's friends or parents as a result of teasing from peers. Because the visual and psychological improvement following the operation is usually dramatic, it is rewarding to the patient, the family, and to the surgeon. The most common reason for prominent ears is excess cartilage. The predisposition to having protruding ears tends to run throughout a family tree and is a dominant trait (so if a parent has it there is a 50% chance the child will). Some family members will have ears that look fairly normal but others will have one or usually both ears that protrude, at least to some degree. The second most common cause is from the top of the ear partially folding over as a result of it missing a piece of cartilage that held it back (lack of the superior crus of the anti-helical fold).

Because the front half of the head develops from two sides that then come together in the middle, rarely are the two ears identical prior to surgery. This is often not noticed because rarely do you see both of the ears at the same time. If the ears are not symmetric to start, chances are there will be some slight differences after the surgery as well. This is cosmetically acceptable because the difference is usually minimal and again, because it is difficult to see both ears simultaneously to compare.

The otoplasty procedure is designed to "complete" the developmental process that failed to completely form all of the folds and crevices in the ear. This is done by positioning the ears closer to the head and attempting to recreate the folds by placing sutures and shaping the cartilage in the ear so that they can "heal" in their desired position.

In children, the surgery is preferably done before they begin school, to avoid classroom teasing and "nicknames," but it can be done at any age after 2. By the age of six (6) the ears have reached about 90 percent of their adult size, so little growth occurs after this time. Studies have shown that operating younger than this does not cause any problems with the growth of the ear so you should feel comfortable having your child undergo the surgery.

When the ear cartilage is thick and strong, it tends to resist being repositioned and a "tuck-up" procedure might be indicated within 6-12 months. This is more common in older children and adults as the cartilages in the ear tend to become firmer with age.

Even if only one ear appears to protrude excessively, it is not uncommon to correct both to differing degrees in order to attain the desired surgical result.

## The Surgery

In younger children, this is best performed using a general anesthetic at the hospital or outpatient surgical centers. Without the appropriate degree of anesthesia children tend to not be willing participants for a delicate surgery. In adults and older children, the procedure can be performed in the clinic with local anesthesia. The procedure is usually performed as an outpatient procedure provided a responsible adult can look after the patient. In most cases there is minimal pain after this type of surgery. Anything more than minimal pain needs to be brought to my attention immediately as it could be the sign of a developing problem.

There are two ways of performing otoplasty. One involves an incision behind the ear and one is the incisionless technique. Most commonly I perform the incisionless technique as this allows for quicker healing and less risk. If an incision is made, the scars resulting from the surgical incisions are located behind each ear and are hidden in the creases. It is rare for these scars to thicken or hypertrophy. If this should happen, they can usually be softened with steroid injections.

A turban-type bandage is worn about the head to cover the ears the night after surgery. After this bandage is removed, (usually the next morning), the patient wears a stocking cap or head band pulled down over the ears for another week and while sleeping for one month. Most patients may return to work or school in 5-7 days following surgery or sooner depending on the type of work performed.

The sutures used to close the skin incisions behind the ears, if used, usually dissolve. Do not pull the ears forward under any circumstances as this can ruin the entire operation! With the incisionless technique the ears cannot get wet for one week. The use of any force or rubbing over the ear can ruin the results as well.

When the dressings are first removed, your ears will appear to have been over corrected or too close to the head. In time they begin to assume their new position. With any surgery, it takes time for healing to be complete, so do not try to evaluate the results too early. We want to monitor the healing, so please keep the post-operative appointments. On rare occasions, one of the deeper sutures may work its way to the skin surface. If this happens a small procedure under local anesthesia can be used to replace the suture.

## After Otoplasty

The following are designed to answer practically every question that may arise regarding the "dos" and "don'ts" after surgery. You and your family should read the instructions several times to familiarize yourselves thoroughly with them. Attempt to follow them faithfully, because those who do so generally have the smoothest post-operative course. This, of course, favors proper healing and a better result. Failure to follow these instructions faithfully can lead to certain complications which potentially could jeopardize the desired result.

### Post-Operative Instructions for Open Otoplasty

DO: Clean your incisions with hydrogen peroxide six (6) times daily and then place the antibiotic ointment in a fine line around the incisions.
DO: Keep the head band on at all times except when showering for the first week.
DO: Report any increasing pain or sudden swelling immediately to us.

* * * * *

DO NOT: Sleep on your side as this can put pressure on the stitches
DO NOT: Pull on your ears to look at them as this can ruin the entire surgery.

### Remember the things you were told before your operation, namely:

1. Sleep on your back and use your head band
2. It is ok to take a shower the day after surgery and get the area wet but do NOT rub your ears. Pat off the drippy water and allow them to air dry.
3. Your ears will appear swollen initially. Do not begin to judge the results until 2 weeks after surgery. In the beginning, we are only evaluating the healing process.
4. If there is any sudden worsening in pain or ear swelling, contact us immediately.
5. Avoid any strenuous activity for the first two (2) weeks after surgery. After this you can begin to initiate your previous activity, but listen to your body.
6. Avoid any contact sports for two (2) months. Keep in mind that any direct trauma to the ears such as that which occurs in wrestling can reverse many of the changes that had been created surgically.
7. Most patients can return to school seven (7) days after surgery. Your ears will likely still be swollen and discolored at this time and you will still be wearing your headband. By two (2) weeks most of this will have gone away.
8. When you should return to work depends on the amount of physical activity and public contact your job involves, in addition to the amount of swelling and discoloration you develop. The average patient may return to work by the seventh to tenth postoperative day, some sooner.

### Report to the Clinic Any:

1. Temperature elevation greater than 100 degrees
2. Sudden swelling or discoloration.
3. Hemorrhage.
4. Discharge from the wound edges or other evidence of infection.
5. Development of any reaction to medications.
6. Sudden worsening of pain

If you have any questions call

832-956-1040

# Chapter 9

## Surgery of the Eyelids

**Blepharoplasty**

**No-Scar Lower Lid Surgery: Trans conjunctival Blepharoplasty**

**Classical Lower Lid Surgery**

**Fat Repositioning**

**The Other "Bulge"**

**After Eyelid Surgery**

*Swelling and Discoloration*
*Your Medications*
*Hemorrhage*
*Temperature*
*Post-Operative Clinic Visits*
*The Healing Period*
*Post-Operative Instructions*
*Remember the things you were told before your operation, namely*
*Report to the Clinic Any*

# Blepharoplasty

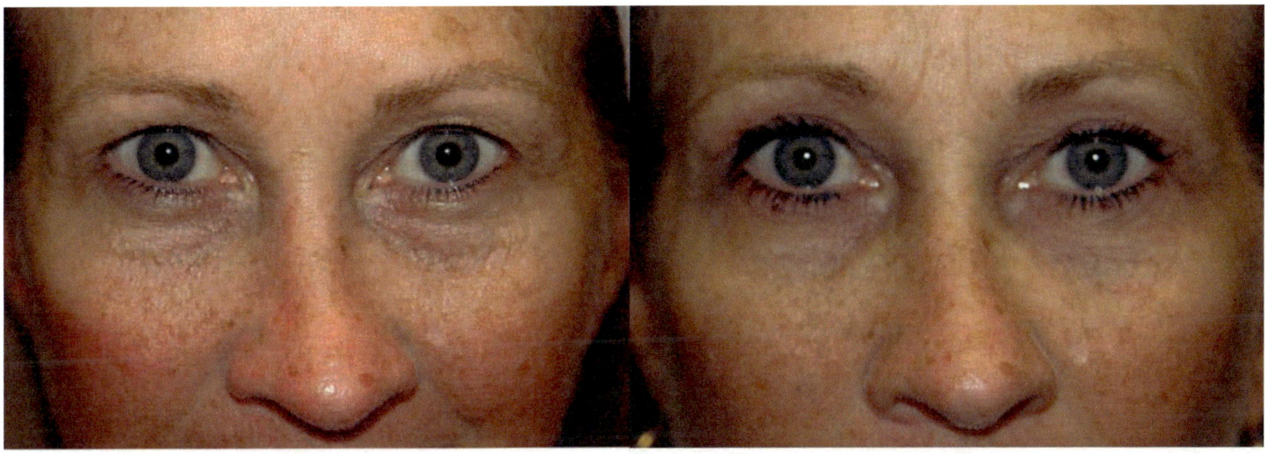

Before After

This patient, in her 50s, is 2 weeks out following an upper eyelid blepharoplasty performed under local anesthesia in the Clinic. You can see her lack of swelling and bruising. In fact, most people would not be able to tell she had had surgery only two weeks ago. Notice the improvement in the eyelid skin and how it no longer hangs over her eyelashes. In fact, in the after photo you can see her upper eyelid eyelashes which were nearly completely hidden in the before photo.

Humans have two sets of eyelids—two upper lids and two lower lids. The eyelids function to cleanse the eyes with blinks and protect the eyes from the environment. With age they frequently develop wrinkles, loose or crepey skin, and bulges of fat due either to hereditary factors (seen in younger patients) or the aging process. Pouches or bags of the upper and lower lids are generally due to herniation, or pseudo herniation, of the fat normally localized within the eye socket. There are two of these fat pouches in the upper eyelid and three in the lower eyelid. When you are young, the fat is kept in place by a nice tight membrane. With age, that membrane begins to weaken which allows the fat to protrude. In some patients, these fatty pouches are seen as young as 20, sometimes younger, and can often be corrected at that time. There is little rationale to wait for some arbitrary age before having surgery. When the problem exists, it should be corrected.

Upper eyelid surgery is usually done at the same time as the lower lid surgery, but either can be done as an isolated procedure. Operating only on the upper eyelids is more common than only operating on the lower eyelids, but the patient's preference is followed. Upper and lower eyelid plastic surgery may be performed alone but it is frequently performed with other cosmetic procedures, especially face lifts (Chapter 11) and skin resurfacing procedures (Chapter 12).

In the upper eyelid blepharoplasty, a determination is made about the excess or overlapping skin which frequently obliterates the natural crease above the lashes. In extreme cases, it can even obstruct your vision. After the area has been anesthetized the excess skin and fat are removed and the incision sites are closed with fine sutures.

As a rule, eyelid procedures are

associated with minor discomfort and allow one to return to routine living the following day. Most patients tell us that there is little or no pain in the postoperative period although pain medication will be provided. Each operation is followed by varying degrees of swelling and/or discoloration, most of which usually subsides within 7-10 days. By this time, too, the scars can be camouflaged by makeup. These scars gradually blend in with the surrounding skin after several months and, in most cases, become perceptible only upon close scrutiny.

We recommend you have an eye examination prior to eyelid surgery. Please advise us of any history of eye diseases, dry eyes, the use of eye drops, history of eye infections, or history of visual problems so that we may have them evaluated.

Insurance will not cover surgical fees and hospitalization expenses for cosmetic surgery. However, for patients who have extreme amounts of overhanging tissues producing "hooding," we may request a consultation from an eye specialist. If the examination demonstrates any visual impairment from such a problem, a portion of the fees for "functional" upper lid surgery may be covered by medical insurance.

We have yet to encounter a case where excess skin and fat in the lower lid impaired one's vision; however, if we need to do a procedure to support a lax or drooping lower lid, your insurance may pay some of the costs for this portion of the lower lid operation. No guarantees can ever be made regarding whether your insurance will cover any part of any procedure so you should plan accordingly.

NOTE: At times the curtain of skin hanging from the upper eyelid may be partially or completely due to sagging of the eyebrows. In such cases, it may be necessary to advise elevation and support to the brows and forehead at the same time the upper eyelid plastic surgery is performed (see next section on "The Eyebrow Lift"). If present, it is important to address the sagging eyebrows as well to prevent pulling them down farther by removing only eyelid skin.

## No-Scar Lower Lid Surgery: Transconjunctival Blepharoplasty

In some patients, the herniated fat producing "bags" or bulges in the lower lid can be removed without making an incision in the skin. The incision is made in the pink part behind the lower eyelid, thereby eliminating a visible scar on the skin. But it is not possible to remove loose skin or sagging wrinkles when this method is used. Skin resurfacing (lasers or peeling) can be performed at the same time in order to minimize many of the fine wrinkles, but for patients with a significant amount of extra skin, an external incision is frequently recommended. The transconjunctival surgical approach is usually reserved for younger patients who are afflicted more with the fat herniation than wrinkles or sagging skin.

## Classical Lower Lid Surgery

The lower lid procedure may also be performed by making an incision in the skin below the lower lashes at a level determined by myself. There are two possible locations for this incision: the first is directly below the eyelashes and the second in the first wrinkle. The benefit of just below the eyelashes is the incision is hidden better initially but it carries a much higher risk of having the eyelid fall away from the eyeball (called ectropion). By placing the incision in the first wrinkle below the eyelid this risk is minimized. The scar initially is more noticeable but within a few months the incision lines of both the upper and lower eyelids are essentially non-visible. With either route, the incision is made and the skin elevated so that the fatty pouches or "hernias" can be identified. Once fat is removed, the excess skin is trimmed. Small, delicate sutures are used to close the lower lid incisions. When loose skin needs to be removed it is necessary to make the incision on the outside of the lid. Because the skin at the outer corners of the eye is thicker than the skin adjacent to the lashes, it takes a little longer for that area to soften and flatten after surgery. If needed, steroid injections can speed the process along.

## Fat Repositioning

Fat repositioning is the process used in lower eyelid surgery to help improve the appearance of a prominent tear trough. The tear trough is the area between the lower eyelid and the nose. In some patients, this can become hollow. A standard lower eyelid blepharoplasty will not improve this area. Instead, a portion of the excess fat that would otherwise be removed is repositioned to the tear trough area to help smooth it out and provide for a more natural transition between the eyelid and the nose. This does tend to cause a little more bruising and swelling initially, but when indicated, it can help to provide for a better surgical result.

## The Other "Bulge"

Blepharoplasty is designed to correct conditions found within the confines of the bony rims of the eye socket. This is where the fat is present. Many people ask if lower lid surgery removes or improves the swollen, puffy areas that sometimes develop beneath the lower lid and over the cheek bones. The answer is no. These bulges are thought to be caused by uncontrolled fluid accumulation in the tissues or from allergies. They are essentially "bags of water." Direct excision may remove these unwanted tissues, but this is not indicated unless they become quite large. The resultant scar may be imperceptible, but often requires dermabrasion at a later time to achieve this when the "bulge" is directly excised.

## After Eyelid Surgery

The following are designed to answer practically every question that may arise regarding the "dos" and "don'ts" after surgery. You and your family should read the instructions several times to familiarize yourselves thoroughly with them. Attempt to follow them faithfully, because those who do so generally have the smoothest post-operative course. This, of course, favors proper healing and a better result. Failure to follow these instructions faithfully can lead to certain complications which potentially could jeopardize the desired result. Whenever a question arises, refer back to this book. Chances are you will find the answer, but if you cannot please call us (832-956-1040). If you ever have a concern, call us. It is essential that our staff has the opportunity to evaluate any problem which may arise.

### Swelling and Discoloration

As you were advised before surgery, a varying amount of swelling and discoloration follows every one of these operations, so try not to become anxious or depressed about it as the swelling will pass. However, healing takes longer in some patients than in others. If you consider yourself a person who bruises easily, chances are you will have a little more bruising than someone who doesn't bruise easily We try to keep swelling to a minimum by limiting any medications preoperatively that may thin the blood and by using meticulous surgical techniques.

The intermittent application of cold compresses 20 minutes of each waking hour for the first three (3) days following surgery is very helpful. After that it probably doesn't help, but some people still find it soothing and it is okay to continue. The important thing to remember is they are cold compresses, NOT ice compresses. Never put anything taken out of your freezer directly on your skin. After surgery, the skin may be numb temporarily and not feel the damage or frostbite occurring from ice placed directly on the skin. If you use cold compresses more frequently than above it can also cause your skin to become pink and irritated.

In the immediate period after surgery, we are evaluating the healing process. Do not attempt to evaluate the results of your surgery while the tissues are swollen. Although you will see some immediate improvement, things look better when the swelling has dissipated. It may take a few months to see your final result, but you will have a good idea how things will look within a few weeks.

### Your Medications

When you are discharged after surgery you should already have several prescriptions. These will include an antibiotic, a pain pill, and a sleeping pill. Because this type of surgery is rarely painful, the pain medication should be used only if the cold compresses do not suffice. This is because pain relievers other than acetaminophen (Tylenol) usually cause sensations of dizziness or drowsiness and make recovery more tedious. If you continue to have discomfort, it is okay to take the prescribed pain medication as directed. The other prescription will be for insomnia. Take it if you have difficulty falling asleep at night as directed. Also, make sure not to take your sleeping pill within 2 hours of taking your prescription pain pill. Some people need only a combination of acetaminophen (Tylenol ®) and diphenhydramine (Benadryl®) in a single pill called Percogesic ® which can be purchased without a prescription to help them both with pain and sleep. Finally, an eye lubricating ointment is provided to be placed on the incision line to keep it moist as described below.

### Hemorrhage

If any prominent bleeding occurs lay down, elevate your head, apply cold compresses over your eyes, and have someone report it to us by telephone immediately. It is normal to have a very minimal amount of blood-tinged drainage around the wounds.

However, notify us immediately of any sudden swelling or change in vision as this could represent a very rare but serious issue.

### Temperature

Generally, the body temperature does not rise much above 100 degrees following eyelid surgery. This rise is usually due to dehydration caused by an insufficient intake of fluids. People often think they have an increased temperature because they feel warm, when, in reality, they may not. To be sure you have a fever, measure your temperature with a thermometer and report any persistent temperature above 100 degrees.

### Post-Operative Clinic Visits

Upon discharge, you should confirm your next appointment.

Don't build up a feeling of fear and anxiety about what is going to be done during this visit. A few skin sutures may require removal; however, many of the sutures used in eyelid surgery dissolve with the peroxide and ointment treatments and do not require removal. The incisions will be gently cleansed and you will probably feel much better. Most patients don't even feel the sutures being removed.

### The Healing Period

1. Swelling may sometimes persist longer than usual. The same is true of discoloration. This is more common in patients who tend to "bruise easily." Both the swelling and discoloration generally reach their peak on the second to fourth post-operative day, so do not become alarmed. In some patients, there is hardly any swelling or discoloration. Furthermore, if you have nasal allergies or "sinus trouble," you should take antihistamines as this may be a contributing factor to swelling about the eyes.
2. Rarely, the whites of one or both eyes may become partially discolored. This is painless and usually absorbs within a week or so. If disconcerting, an eye drop may be prescribed to speed up this process.
3. Occasionally, swelling will cause the lower lid to be separated from the eyeball. This condition should reverse as the swelling subsides, but it can be prolonged if face powder, granules, etc., become deposited in the area when cosmetics are being applied. Notify us if it persists. If the eyes feel "dry" use artificial tears or other nonprescription eye lubricants as needed.
4. During the first several days following surgery, the scars may be imperceptible. They then go through a period of swelling, become red or deep pink in color, and develop some lumpiness especially at the outer corners. This is part of the healing process and eventually subsides. As time passes, they should once again become virtually imperceptible. This is the way scars normally "mature." Thus, any unevenness of the edges of the incisions or lumpiness of the scars is usually temporary and subsides with the passage of time. Cosmetics or steroid injections may be used to minimize the visibility of the lumps while progressive maturation of the scars is occurring. Remember, maturation takes longer in the thicker skin of the outer corners. Minor revisions can be performed if necessary. We will suggest them, if appropriate.
5. Occasionally, small cysts which resemble "whiteheads" may appear within the lid incision sites. They are

blocked oil glands. They should disappear after their contents are expressed. They may occur in both the upper and lower lids.

6. Patients often experience some blurring of vision for two (2) or three (3) days after the operation. This is generally due to swelling and/or ointments that have been used and should clear spontaneously. Notify us however if you are concerned or of any change in your vision.

### Post-Operative Instructions

Please follow these instructions carefully. You should also review the materials in the consultation book relative to your surgery. Your final result will depend upon how well you care for the treated areas.

DO: Clean suture lines with hydrogen peroxide and a Q-tip as directed.

DO: Apply the provided ophthalmic ointment to sutures following cleaning.

DO: Apply the ophthalmic ointment or moisturizing drops in your eyes if they feel dry or irritated.

DO: Report any eye pain or change in your vision to the clinic staff immediately.

DO: Wear glasses, if necessary, making sure they do not pull on incision lines.

DO: Continue cold compresses over your eyelids for at least 24 hours and preferably up to 3 days.

DO: Sleep with your head elevated 30 to 40 degrees for ideally 2 weeks.

DO: Wash your hair following surgery if desired.

* * * * *

DO NOT: Apply any makeup (mascara, eyeliner or eye shadow) for the first 10 days following surgery and never to resurfaced areas until directed to do so.

DO NOT: Wear contact lenses for 10 days.

DO NOT: Pluck eyebrows for 2 weeks.

**Remember the things you were told before your operation, namely:**

1. Continue to take the prescribed medications and antibiotics until your supply is exhausted; these prescriptions need not be refilled. Take pain and sleeping medications as needed and directed.
2. Sleep with your head elevated 30 to 40 degrees for ideally 2 weeks. This is best accomplished with the use a recliner.
3. Apply cold compresses made of face towels (not an ice bag).
4. STAY UP (sitting, standing, walking around) after the day of surgery! Of course, you should rest when you tire and don't do anything that elevates your heart rate.
5. Avoid bending over or lifting heavy objects for two (2) weeks. Besides aggravating swelling, this may raise the blood pressure and start a hemorrhage.
6. Avoid straining when going to the bathroom, which also raises the blood pressure. If you feel you need a laxative, take one you are accustomed to using. Prescription pain medications sometimes cause constipation so use them sparingly.
7. Avoid hitting and bumping your face and eyes. It is wise not to pick up small children who often move unexpectedly. You should sleep alone for one (1) week after your operation to avoid inadvertent bumping by a sleeping partner.
8. Avoid excessive sunning of the face for prolonged periods during the first thirty (30) days following the operation. Ordinary sun exposure as part of your usual day is not harmful.

9. Don't pluck your eyebrows for two (2) weeks.
10. You may gently shampoo your hair 24 hours after your surgery. Water and shampoo will not ordinarily harm the incisions. If you need to blow dry your hair, use a blow dryer set on a cool setting for the first two (2) post-operative weeks.
11. You may take a shower the day after surgery. Do not be afraid to get the suture lines wet. If you had skin resurfacing, follow the instructions pertaining to those procedures.
12. If you have had incisions into the skin of the eyelids, go over your suture lines as directed with a Q-tip saturated with full strength hydrogen peroxide, but avoid getting any in your eyes. Then put a very small amount of the recommended ophthalmic lubricating ointment on a Q-tip and apply it to the suture lines. Avoid getting too much in your eyes, as it may cause blurring of the vision or irritation. Do not use the antibiotic ointment prescribed for other sutures lines if you underwent multiple procedures. Do not let Q-tips or ointments come in contact with resurfaced areas.
13. Take only prescribed pain relievers or non-aspirin pain relievers such as Tylenol ® but never aspirin or ibuprofen as they promote bleeding.
14. Report any bleeding that persists after holding gentle pressure for 15-20 minutes.
15. Notify us immediately of any sudden swelling or change in your vision.
16. You may begin wearing eyeglasses or sun glasses the day following eyelid surgery. Do not put your contact lenses in for at least ten (10) days and only after you have received approval from us.
17. Don't swim, dive, ski, or participate in strenuous athletic activity for at least two (2) weeks after surgery.
18. Eye shadow and false eyelashes should not be applied until about ten (10) days after surgery. Again, clear this with us prior to use.
19. You can camouflage the discoloration about the eyes with makeup before you come to the Clinic to get your first set of sutures removed unless resurfacing was also performed. Do not apply makeup over any of your incisions. Bring it near the incision line but do not apply over the incisions themselves until two (2) days after the sutures have been removed.
20. You should not plan to return to work until a few days have elapsed following the surgery. Even then, it might be wise to procure sunglasses with large frames unless you don't mind the extra attention.

**Report to The Clinic Any:**

1. Temperature elevation greater than 100 degrees
2. Sudden swelling or discoloration.
3. Hemorrhage.
4. Discharge from the wound edges or other evidence of infection.
5. Development of any reaction to medications.

If you have any questions call

832-956-1040

# Chapter 10

## Surgery of the Eyebrows

**The Eyebrow Lift**

**Surgical Options**

**After Eyebrow Lift Surgery**

*Post-Operative Instructions*

*Remember the things you were told before your operation, namely*

*Report to the Clinic Any*

## The Eyebrow Lift

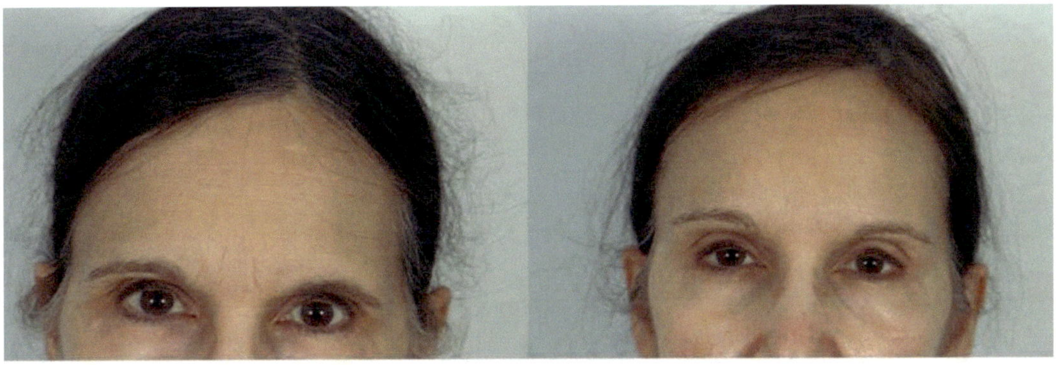

Before DR. GUY FACIAL PLASTIC SURGERY After

> This patient in her early 60s was bothered by the heaviness of her brows. They were creating an angry face. She could raise her brows up with her forehead muscle but this created forehead wrinkles. Therefore, we treated her with an endoscopic brow lift. This utilizes four little access holes within the hairline and surgically raises the eyebrow. You can see in the after photo taken at 6 months post operatively how much more open her eyes are, even though the eyelids themselves were not changed. This shows what a brow lift can accomplish with minimal downtime.

Drooping of the eyebrows is frequently one of the first signs of aging. The reason is anatomy. There is no muscle or structure that pulls up the outer corner of the eyebrows, but there is a muscle that pulls them down. This downward pulling muscle is the one that goes all the way around the eye so every time you smile or close your eyes, you are pulling down on your eyebrows. This condition is often overlooked because most people are unaware of the problem and the degree of improvement its correction can provide.

A heavy eyebrow causes the upper eyelids to drop or descend until, in the advanced stages, eyelid skin can touch or overlap the eyelashes. Patients often complain that their eyes appear to be getting smaller or deeper-set and that eye make-up usually ends up high on the upper part of the lids within a short while after it has been applied. Drooping eyebrows definitely contribute to the "tired look." When the inside of the eyebrows begins to droop, which happens with more advanced age, it contributes to an "angry look."

# Surgical Options

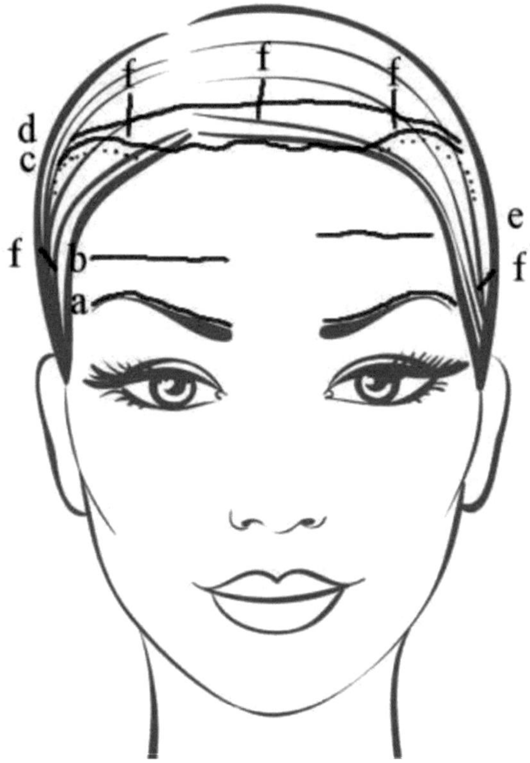


This picture shows the multiple incision options for a brow lift as described below.

a) Direct
b) Mid forehead
c) Pretrichial
d) Coronal
e) Temporal (dashed)
f) Endoscopic

There are multiple techniques to raise the eyebrows. Some are better for certain conditions and patients. The first way is known as the direct brow lift. This involves an incision directly above your eyebrow. The benefit of this technique is it allows the brows to be elevated independently to help with any asymmetry or differences between the two sides. There is also no numbness on the top of the scalp. The drawback is the incision and resulting scar is visible although it is camouflaged between the forehead and the eyebrow to help. This method is usually reserved for patients with a facial paralysis or in males with a lot of redundant skin with droopy eyebrows causing visual obstruction. It can also be done under local anesthesia in the office.

The next approach is one step higher than the direct approach. It is called the indirect approach or mid-forehead lift. The incision for this is placed into a natural crease on the forehead. The benefit is this can also help with asymmetry between the brows. It is reserved for patients with very deep creases in the forehead which allow the scar to be camouflaged. This is usually reserved for males who have a receding hairline and deep creases that could camouflage the incision. It can also be done under local anesthesia in the office.

The next two approaches are similar. The first is known as the pretrichial incision or the "in front of the hairline" incision. The incision is made just in front of the hairline, beveled in such a way that it allows the hairs to grow through the scar to camouflage it. This method not only raises the eyebrows but also can help to lower an otherwise high forehead. There is commonly numbness of the crown which can be permanent. The second of these approaches is the coronal incision. It is placed a few centimeters (about an inch) behind the hairline. The benefit is that the scar is camouflaged, but it does raise the forehead as well. It is also associated with numbness of the scalp. There is also the risk of hair loss on both sides of the incision. These are approaches that are commonly performed on females or males without a receding hairline who could also benefit from raising the inside of the eyebrow. They can also be done under local anesthesia in the office but more commonly are performed in the operating room.

The temporal approach is a modification of the pretrichial and coronal approaches. It helps raise the outer portion of the eyebrows. This incision is made entirely within the hairline and can be used in receding hairlines to some extent. It can be associated with numbness but not often. It is frequently utilized as part of a cheek lift in order to improve the appearance of the outside part of the eye as well.

The last approach is known as the endoscopic approach. This involves making several small incisions within your hairline, and then using a tiny camera to help raise your eyebrows. The eyebrows are then secured in their new position with sutures. The benefit of this approach is there are no visible incisions and it is less invasive than the other options. This is the most common choice for those who have heavy inside and outside corners of the brow. Since no skin is removed with this incision, for the first few weeks it will appear like you have "carpet rolls" behind the small incisions. This represents how much skin was elevated. Over the course of a few weeks to rarely a few months this will flatten out as the redundant skin tightens up. This method is very useful for those with lesser degrees of brow ptosis and those who don't want any external scars. It also is the least likely to cause prolonged scalp numbness.

All of these techniques "lift" the brow, upper lid to some extent, and surrounding tissues which usually results in eyes that appear larger, more rested and more youthful. There is often lessening of the deeper "crow's feet" found next to the outer corners of the eye. However, for the best result, "crow's feet" may require a skin resurfacing procedure either at the same time or at a later date.

The eyebrow lift will not correct either excess skin or bulges caused by fat herniation at the inner corners of the upper eyelids, and it will not have any effect on lower lid conditions. On the other hand, it can be, and often is, effectively combined with eyelid surgery (Chapter 9).

Frequently the brow lift is accompanied by a face lift (Chapter 11), but it may be performed as an independent procedure.

## After Eyebrow Lift Surgery

The following are designed to answer practically every question that may arise regarding the "dos" and "don'ts" after surgery. You and your family should read the instructions several times to familiarize yourselves thoroughly with them. Attempt to follow them faithfully, because those who do so generally have the smoothest post-operative course. This, of course, favors proper healing and a better result. Failure to follow these instructions faithfully can lead to certain complications which potentially could jeopardize the desired result.

Whenever a question arises, refer

back to this book. Chances are you will find the answer, but if you cannot please call us (832-956-1040). If you ever have a concern, call us. It is essential that our staff has the opportunity to evaluate any problem which may arise.

### Post-Operative Instructions

Please follow these instructions carefully. You should also review the materials in the consultation book relative to your surgery. Your final result will depend upon how well you care for the treated areas.

DO: For non-hair bearing incisions, Clean suture lines with hydrogen peroxide and a Q-tip as directed. For sutures within the hairline use Witch Hazel instead of hydrogen peroxide to prevent bleaching of your roots.

DO: Take all medications as prescribed. Only take the prescription pain medication if needed as it can lead to sleepiness and make the recovery period more uncomfortable. For more mild pain, use either Tylenol ® as instructed.

DO: Apply the antibiotic ointment over all non-hair bearing incisions after cleaning except the ones within the hairline. If tape was placed over your incisions, you do not need to clean them or apply ointment to them.

DO: Take a shower the day after surgery using water only with no shampoo or soap.

DO: Take a shower the second day after surgery using shampoo.

DO: Continue cold compresses over the forehead for 3 days.

DO: Sleep with your head elevated 30 to 40 degrees to minimize swelling for at least two (2) weeks and preferably four (4) weeks.

DO: Stay upright as much as possible to help the swelling go away faster.

DO: Begin walking on the second post-operative day.

* * * * *

DO NOT: Use hot water for showering as you may have numbness of your scalp.

DO NOT: Use a hair dryer unless it is on setting COLD or COOL.

DO NOT: Pluck eyebrows for two (2) weeks.

DO NOT: Engage in any activity that involves raising your blood pressure or bending over as this can lead to bleeding and affect your final result.

DO NOT: Jog for four (4) weeks after surgery.

### Remember the things you were told before your operation, namely:

1. The day after surgery let warm water run through the hair while standing in a shower. Two (2) days after surgery you may use a recommended shampoo. If you had eyelid surgery, do not be afraid to get the sutures around your eyes wet when showering. You should shampoo at least daily for the first post-operative week.
2. Numbness on the top of your head is normal. Do not itch or scratch the top of the head in order to prevent hair loss. If you have an itch, use a single finger to push on the area and the itch will go away.
3. Report any bleeding that persists after steady pressure has been held on the area for twenty (20) minutes or report immediately any profuse bleeding, although this is exceptionally rare.
4. Report any sudden swelling of your forehead.

5. Report any of the warning signs of an infection such as sudden or excessive localized swelling, redness, drainage, or fever.
6. Avoid taking medications on an empty stomach as they may produce nausea. Some medications, especially antibiotics, can produce digestive system upset. Please notify us if you have a problem. We can usually prescribe another one for you.
7. Never wash your hair the day that sutures, clips or staples are removed. Wash it the following day.
8. Hair sprays, conditioners and vegetable color rinses (Roux®) can be used in two (2) weeks.
9. Avoid lifting your eyebrows for two weeks. If you continuously try to raise and lower your eyebrows you may widen your scars and affect the final position of your eyebrows. For the endoscopic approach, you can dislodge the skin off of the absorbable implant and lose your lift.
10. If your eyebrows are taped up for the first week, do not pull on the tape as they are there to help the healing process.
11. Make sure you keep all post-operative appointments.

**Report To The Clinic Any:**

1. Temperature elevation greater than 100 degrees
2. Sudden swelling or discoloration.
3. Hemorrhage.
4. Discharge from the wound edges or other evidence of infection.
5. Development of any reaction to medications.

If you have any questions call 832-956-1040

# Chapter 11

## Surgery of the Aging Face

**The Face Lift Operation: Foreheads, Cheeks, and Necks**

**How Long Does It Last?**

**Who Should Have a Face Lift?**

**Must I Have Another Face lift?**

**When is Facial Plastic Surgery Indicated?**

**Why Does the Face Droop and Sag?**

**Should I Lose Weight Before Surgery?**

**Will Surgery Correct Laugh and Frown Lines?**

**The Problem Neck: Facial and Neck Liposuction and Submental Lipectomy**

**About The Surgery**

**Why do some people not look like "themselves" after face lifting surgery?**

**Incisions and Scars**

**After Face Lift Surgery**

*Swelling*
*Discoloration*
*Turning the Head*
*Discomfort*
*Ice Compresses*
*Removal of Dressings*
*Elevate the Head of Bed*
*Getting Out of Bed*
*Hemorrhage*
*Temperature*
*Weakness*
*Insomnia*
*Depression*
*Numbness*
*Tightness of the Face*
*Thinning of the Hair*
*If You Injure Your Face*
*Your Medications*
*Resuming Activities*
*Your Scars*
*Follow-up Clinic Visits*
*Post-Operative Instructions*

## The Face Lift Operation: Foreheads, Cheeks, and Necks

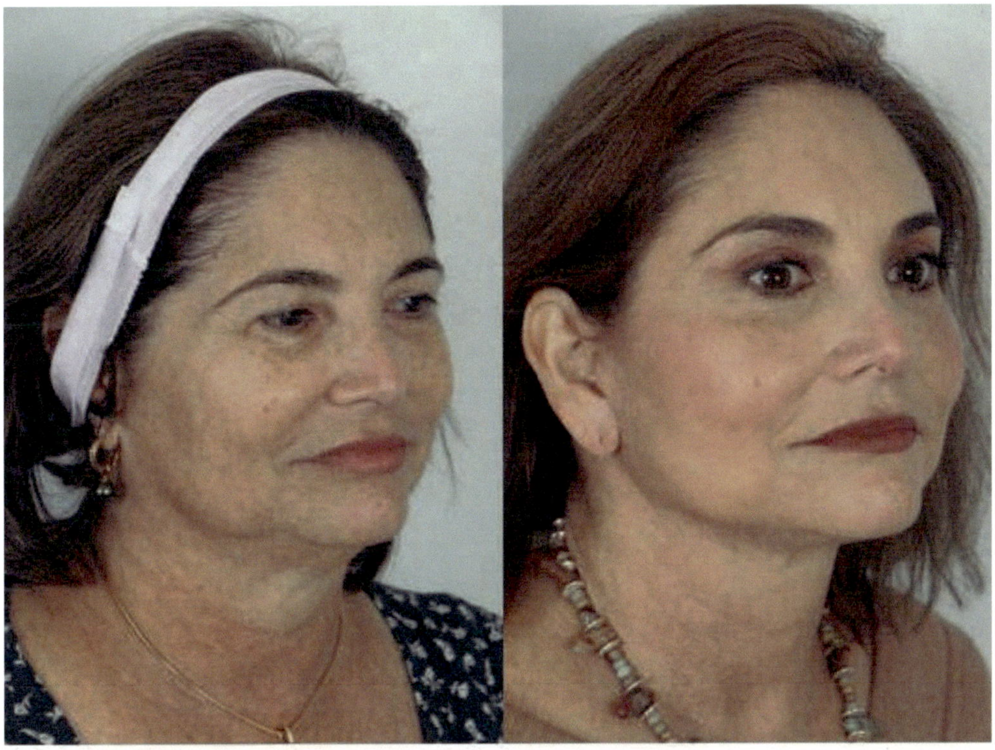

Before DR. GUY After
FACIAL PLASTIC SURGERY

This patient in her early 60s was wanting full face rejuvenation. She wanted to look on the outside how great she felt on the inside. Dr. Guy performed a traditional cheek and neck lift, endoscopic brow lift, upper blepharoplasty (eyelid surgery), lower blepharoplasty, and platysmaplasty with removal of post platysmal fat. In the after photos, taken 4 months post operatively you can see how all of this came together to create a much more youthful appearance. Her jowls are gone. Her neck line is crisp. Her eyes are open and awake. Most importantly, she is ecstatic with the results. Additionally, nothing about her looks “done” as Dr. Guy creates a very natural, rejuvenated result.

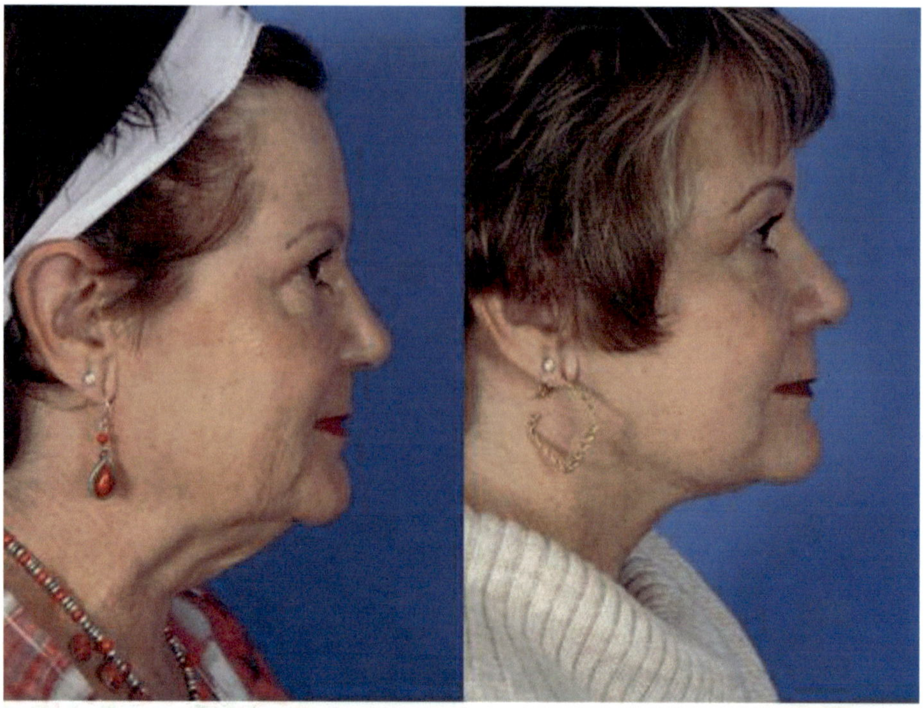

Before DR. GUY FACIAL PLASTIC SURGERY After

This patient in her late 60s was bothered by how her neck and face aged her. Dr. Guy performed a deep plane cheek and neck lift with platsymaplasty, liposuction, and upper and lower blepharoplasty (eyelid surgery). In the after photo, you can see how improved her neck and jowls are, how she has a jawline, and how much more youthful she looks. Most importantly she still looks like herself, just a younger version.

The Greek word for wrinkle is "rhytid." The suffix -ectomy means "to remove." Thus, rhytidectomy is the medical term for the operation designed to remove or lift wrinkles and sagging tissues from the forehead, face, and neck. The term "face lift" is often used incorrectly in the media. This may be to help market some new fad or it can be used to describe a total facial rejuvenation, which, in reality, consists of an eyelid surgery, a face lift, and possibly skin resurfacing. While a true face lift provides the foundation for the rejuvenation process, other procedures may add the finishing touches. By no means, however, does this mean that every patient who requests a face lift should have any additional procedures. These are only recommended if they would provide further benefit, and if the patient is interested in these procedures.

Face lifting may be done for one or two reasons: to help prevent the advancement of aging, i.e., to help relatively young individuals (about 40 or less) to appear to stay young. The second reason is to assist one who is already showing more advanced signs of aging or whose skin sags to appear younger and more rested.

The goal of the face lift operation is to reduce the signs of aging. In the face, these manifest as alternating ridges/bulges and hollows with each bulge having previously filled in the hollow above it. With time, the once full and youthful face begins to sag and the skin loosens. A face lift is deigned to counteract these forces by lifting the tissues and restoring them to their more youthful position. This includes not only lifting the skin but more importantly the underlying muscles and fatty tissues. It is important to realize that a face lift does not correct problems in the upper or lower eyelids, or the wrinkles or creases in the lips—other procedures (blepharoplasty, skin resurfacing, and/or lip enhancement) are required for these conditions. The folds extending from the nose to the lateral corners of the lips may be improved but not eliminated with a facelift. They can be further improved by using your own collagen as a filler in this area (Chapter 12) or with fat transfer. How-ever, not all face lifts are the same – nor should they be! The reason is that not all faces are the same. And, at different ages, the same person has different conditions of aging that develop. The facts are plastic surgery is very much an art form and can be tailored by an experienced surgeon/artist to meet the needs of each individual who presents for treatment.

The face lift has become one of the most popular cosmetic operations performed in the head and neck because as medical advances and new technology increase the average life span, many women and men, find that they look older than they feel. The antiquated stigma previously associated with having plastic surgery is disappearing. Men and women from all walks of life are seeking ways to look as good as they feel. The techniques I use produce results which result in "natural" and "un-operated" looks as can be seen in the examples above.

The operation itself may be divided into three parts: the forehead or eyebrow lift (the upper one-third), the cheek lift (the middle one-third), and the neck lift (the lower one-third). Most people require all three components but occasionally only one or two portions are needed or recommended. The most common isolated request is a "neck lift." Most people seeking "neck lifts" require some lifting of the cheeks in order to avoid "puckering" of the skin around the ears. In select patients, it is possible that a neck lift is all that is required. I will recommend what would be of benefit during your consultation.

## How Long Does It Last?

Naturally, everyone contemplating an operation is interested in how much improvement he or she can expect and for what duration. The amount of improvement depends on the degree of wrinkling and sagging present. If it is excessive, the results may be dramatic. If sagging is occurring prematurely and the operation is being done to attempt to keep the patient looking young, the improvement may be more subtle which is the goal of a preventative operation. Frequent comments we hear post-operatively include that the person appears "less tired" and the face "looks more alive, rested and refreshed." Some people look as though they have "lost weight" because the heaviness along the jaw line and in the neck is improved.

Cosmetic surgery turns back the clock but it does not stop the ticking. No operation can permanently prevent aging, but the individual who has undergone surgery to reverse the signs of aging should never appear as old as he/she might have if the operation had not been done. It is as though one's appearance is moved several years back on the "conveyor belt of time." The duration of the results achieved with a face and neck lift cannot always be predicted. In general, the surgery helps turn back the clock about 10 to 15 years in most patients. The excess skin and fat in the neck and lower jaw is removed during surgery and the underlying tissue tightened. These changes are permanent but the moment the surgery ends, time and the aging process continue. If wrinkling and sagging was severe it will take years before the condition becomes as bad as it was before surgery. When the signs of aging do return, this is precisely when a "tuck-up" procedure is helpful. No matter how snugly skin and underlying tissues are drawn, in time they will loosen. And it is impossible to predict when—and to what extent—this may happen. Genetics, age differences, ethnic backgrounds, stress, illness, nutrition, etc., all play a role in how soon "tuck-up" procedures may be considered. This fact is beyond the control of the surgeon.

For the best results, every patient should be evaluated within a year or two following surgery. A "tuck-up" may or may not be discussed at this time. A face lift simply removes the slack which occurred due to the breaking down of the elastic tissues in the skin as part of the aging process; however, like any material that has elasticity, a second tightening may be helpful. The foundation created by the initial face lift creates the desired situation for a "tuck-up." It is not necessary, however, to have additional cosmetic surgery. The "tuck-up" is simply part of a maintenance program. When the original face lift was performed by us and the proper foundation was created, tuck-ups are generally less extensive, less expensive, and quite effective since at this point most of the "slack" of the skin has been removed. This leads to results that tend to last longer.

Claims that some surgeon's face lifts, "last longer" should be viewed with skepticism. "Over-doing" surgery in an attempt to have a "tight" appearance for a longer time is fraught with problems including unnatural and "plastic" looks.

## Who Should Have a Face Lift?

Men and women from all walks of life are having face lifts; however, not everyone seeking improvement is an acceptable candidate for surgery. Those with known serious medical problems may not be surgical candidates depending on the condition and how well it is under control. Patients who are obese with a short, thick, neck have little chance for a worthwhile result. The severe "turkey gobbler" deformity which occurs in the neck of some individuals may best be corrected by a direct excision in the midline of the neck under the chin. Finally, those with unrealistic expectations are not acceptable surgical candidates.

Nicotine interferes with blood flow through the skin of the face, delays healing and tends to increase the incidence of complications by a factor of 17! Please notify us of any tobacco use or smoking cessation aids you may be using. Doing so will be in your best interest and will help to determine the extent of surgery that can be performed.

Each individual who wants to look "better" presents a different set of problems. Consequently, the corrective procedures indicated vary with each case. For example, one person may require only elevation of sagging eyebrows or improvement in the eyelids. A very young individual may need only correction of an early double-chin with liposuction or submentoplasty. On the other hand, a partial or complete face and neck lift followed by a skin resurfacing procedure may be called for in more advanced cases. Skin resurfacing including a chemical face peel, dermabrasion and/or laser resurfacing procedure may provide the "icing on the cake."

As a rule, a face lift, blepharoplasty, or submental lipectomy improves sags and bulges whereas resurfacing (laser, dermabrasion and chemical peeling) improves wrinkles.

## Must I Have Another Face lift?

Many patients believe that once they have a face lift they must have another, otherwise they will look worse than if they never had the first surgery. This has not been our experience.

It is true that a "tuck-up" at a later date can improve additional sagging that might reappear with the normal aging process, but the patient's excessive skin that was removed at the time of the original surgery never returns. The remaining tissues age by the same natural process that has been occurring since birth.

## When is Facial Plastic Surgery Indicated?

"When the best time for facial cosmetic surgery," is an often-asked question. The best answer is when the slack in the skin of the face and neck or "bags" around the eyes are no longer temporary conditions relieved by rest, or when they become increasingly difficult to camouflage with cosmetics.

There is no magical age when people should be considering surgery, as age is just a number. For some patients, this may be early in life such as correcting nasal deformities after puberty. For others, the right time may not be until the signs of aging have advanced in their 50s and 60s and later. As the life expectancy lengthens in America, most people feel vigorous and energetic long after their appearance begins to deteriorate as a result of advancing age. The emotional impact of looking older than one feels can be disconcerting and facial plastic surgery can bring your looks and how you feel back into harmony.

## Why Does the Face Droop and Sag?

The changes associated with aging do not occur all at once. They happen in a slowly progressive manner, involve all components of the face and body, and at different rates in different people. Patients frequently first become aware of the changes related to aging in their mid-30s which becomes more noticeable over a 2-4-year period in their early forties. They often tell us that it seems as though things were holding up well and seemed to "fall" almost overnight. This is never truer than following a period of prolonged stress which is a known factor to advance the aging process. If you ever question this, think how much the presidents seem to age so rapidly over their terms in office.

With aging, the bones become slightly smaller, some fat is absorbed and other fat sags, and the skin loses much of its elasticity which used to keep it tight. This causes the tissues, particularly in the face and neck, to droop and sag. This phenomenon results in a series of events, including deepening of the lines of facial expression in the forehead and at the sides of the mouth, sagging of the eyebrows which causes the eyes to appear smaller and tired, "crow's feet" form at the corners of the eyes, pouches or jowls develop along the jaw line, and, the well-known "double-chin" develops as a result of a new fatty tissue deposit in this area.

At the same time, the skin also shows its age. In some faces the skin become etched with wrinkles. This frequently occurs in those repetitively exposed to the sun and wind as the damage to the skin is cumulative over your life.

The muscles and tissues around the eyes eventually lose some of their tone so that a portion of the fat normally located inside the orbit around the eye bulges forward, or herniates, to produce the commonly seen "bags." This condition is often seen in younger people before many of the other signs of aging have developed. "Circles" under the eyes may be a result of a shadow falling in the crease between these bags and the cheek.

Finally, because of absorption of tissues in the upper lip and gums, the lips become thinner and the tip of the nose drops causing it to appear larger and longer. Repositioning and supporting the tip of the nose can have dramatic and lasting effects on reversing this telltale sign of the aging process

## Should I Lose Weight Before Surgery?

When someone is overweight, weight loss is always encouraged, not only to improve the appearance but also the health and overall energy. If the patient is committed to losing more than 20 pounds, certainly dramatic changes in the face and body contour might occur. In these individuals, we would recommend waiting for the surgery. Ideally, one should be within 10-15 pounds of his or her realistic weight when surgery is performed. If, however, one plans to lose only 5-10 pounds, the changes would not significantly alter what a face lift is designed to accomplish. Furthermore, we prefer patients be "well-nourished" prior to surgery. Crash diets tend to deplete the body of essential nutrients needed for proper healing and are not recommended before surgery or at any time. Sensible weight loss is always encouraged.

## Will Surgery Correct Laugh and Frown Lines?

Neither surgery nor skin resurfacing can correct wrinkles that occur only during facial expressions. The creases around the eyes produced with smiling, the forehead creases that occur with frowning, and the vertical lines in the upper lip that occur with puckering the lips, are due to the contraction of the muscles of facial expression.

Neuromodulators like Botox, Dysport, and Daxxify can be helpful to improve the conditions that are present with activity. If wrinkles and creases are present at rest then resurfacing the skin with chemical peeling, lasers, and/or dermabrasion may be of help.

## The Problem Neck: Facial and Neck Liposuction and Submental Lipectomy/ Submentoplasty

With youth, there is a taught muscle that helps to keep the neck appearing young. With time, this muscle sling weakens, and in most people loose skin and fat are gradually deposited until the so-called "double-chin" develops. This hanging pouch of fat and skin obliterates the ideal angle of the chin-neck profile and contributes to the appearance of aging. Other people develop a "turkey-gobbler" deformity which consists of vertical bands of loose skin and muscle extending from the chin to the base of the neck. Some double-chins may be improved by a procedure known liposuction wherein a small incision is made under the chin, the excess fat is removed, and the skin of the upper part of the neck is tightened as part of a cheek-neck lift. For younger patients, an isolated submentoplasty with contouring of the deep neck structures may be all that is needed without the traditional lift being performed.

In most cases, there is negligible post-operative discomfort and the scar is camouflaged when it matures. When the condition is extreme, other incisions (i.e., a direct midline neck incision) may be designed in an attempt to obtain a better surgical result. It is rarely possible to do a neck lift without some work in the muscles and cheeks as well.

Submental liposuction and a submentoplasty alone are not sufficient for most people. For younger patients, the skin retains enough elasticity that it can contract after liposuction. Beginning in the mid-30s, the skin loses some of this ability and if a tightening procedure is not performed you can be left with hanging skin in this area which is not desirable. This is particularly true when the face tends to sag along the jaw line at the jowls or when a "turkey gobbler" deformity is present.

## About the Surgery

Technically, the face lift operation consists of repositioning and supporting the sagging skin and the underlying tissues of the face and removing the excess skin and fat.

There are several locations where the incisions can be placed during a face lift. The scars in the hair and around the ear may be camouflaged with the adjacent hair or by the natural creases and folds of the ears. Incisions that are next to hair lines are beveled to allow the hairs to grow through the scar and camouflage it better. The incisions within the hairline are made in such a way to minimize trauma to the surrounding hair. On rare occasions, there may be some thinning of the hair around these incision lines. However, I employ techniques designed to protect and preserve hair and to minimize this risk.

If a temporal or forehead lift is performed, the hairline may be altered. For the temporal extension approach, the incisions are tailored to minimize hairline alterations and avoid the telltale sign of a facelift with a loss of hair above the side burns. Essentially, the operation is "customized" to fit the needs and desires of each patient seeking surgery as discussed in the brow lift section.

During preparation for surgery, we do not shave any hair as it does not assist us and only creates concerns for the patients. Instead, the hair is placed into tiny pigtails to allow me to be able to work around it. Because I close those incisions made in the scalp with small metal clips, it is not necessary to shave the hair. Obviously, the fact that one has had surgery is easier to camouflage when hair shaving is avoided. Another distinct advantage of the metal clip closure is that patients may wash their hair the next day after surgery. As a matter of fact, we recommend daily shampoos following face lift surgery starting on day number two (2) after surgery.

Some degree of tightness, numbness or weakness of surrounding tissues is expected following surgery. It is usually temporary, disappearing as healing progresses. The tightness will increase for the first few days as the swelling increases. This is not an "overdone" surgery but merely the body's response to any surgery. As the swelling dissipates the tight sensation will improve. The numbness is most common in front of and below/behind the ears. If a brow lift was performed, depending on the technique then the scalp may also be numb. As the nerves regenerate it is normal to feel little pings, zings, and itches. This is the body healing and it is important not to itch these areas.

The operation may be done either under local or general anesthesia. I am trained and have operated under both conditions. Certain candidates are better for one type over the other. The final decision as to what type is used will rest with Dr. Guy for safety purposes. More than 99% of the face-lifts we perform are done in outpatient facilities, but even if the surgery is performed in the hospital, patients are usually discharged the following day. If the surgery is performed in an outpatient facility instead of the hospital, the total cost is usually considerably less. These arrangements will be discussed during the consultation and depend on your overall health.

A head bandage is worn the night following surgery and commonly a drain is present. As a result, the head bandage is kept snug for your safety, but it is generally removed the next morning when a much more loose fitting supportive garment is used to help with cold compresses. The face may be swollen and some discoloration may be present. This discoloration usually fades away within about 10-14 days but not before it increases for the first two to three days. Patients can return to most of their "normal routine" within two (2) weeks. But the face and neck may feel "tight" and movement will be restricted. This is to be expected as long as the tissues are swollen.

The patient returns to the Clinic in about a week to have the sutures and clips removed. Makeup may be worn by ten (10) days and he/she should be able to return to work and carefully drive an automobile in fourteen (14) days if work was performed on the neck or in seven (7) days if a neck lift was not performed. Patients must not pull against tightness, lie on their sides or engage in heavy lifting during this time. Doing so can interfere with healing and lead to less than favorable results. Specifically, scars will defend themselves and if you pull against them then the scar will likely widen.

For best results and better scars these activities (other than driving) should be avoided for at least 6 weeks following surgery.

## Why do some people not look like "themselves" after face lifting surgery?

Techniques of face lifting vary greatly from surgeon to surgeon. The "stretched" or "windblown" look generally results from overly aggressive surgery and creates an unnatural appearance in my opinion. My techniques including the deep plane lift are specifically designed to give patients a more natural and un-operated appearance. We say to take a look at a picture of yourself form 10-15 years ago, and that is the result we are going for!

## Incisions and Scars

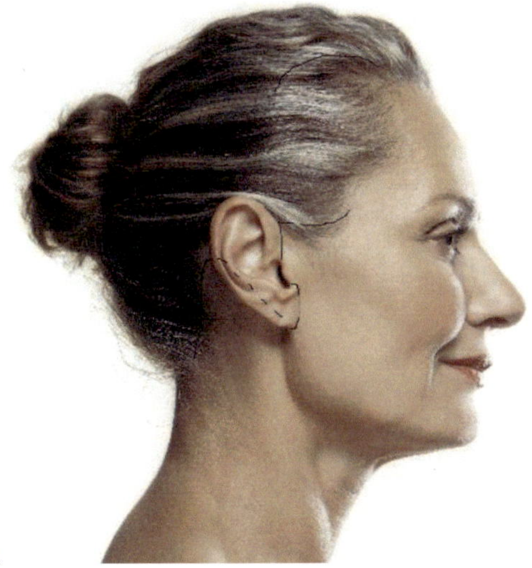

a

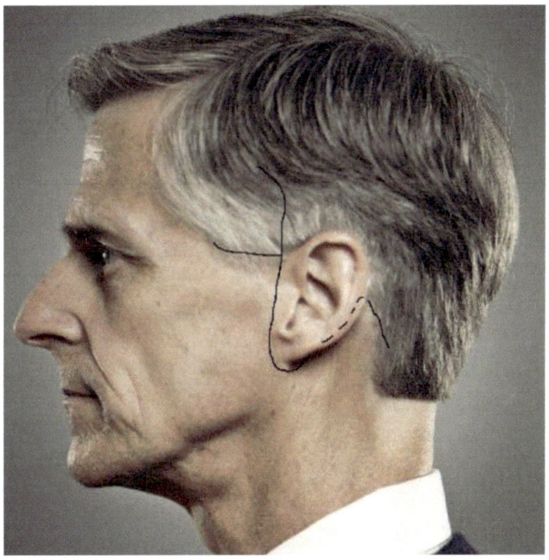

b

a. This photograph demonstrates the usual location of the incisions for a face lift in a woman. They are designed to be camouflaged by the hair and the natural creases around the ear. (The dotted lines indicate the placement of the incisions behind the ear).
b. This photograph demonstrates the typical incisions for a face lift in a man. The pattern of beard growth and the potential for male pattern baldness dictates that the incisions differ from those made in a woman.

Behind the ear the incisions in both men and women are similar. They are usually camouflaged by the natural creases and by the hair.

## After Face Lift Surgery

The following are designed to answer practically every question that may arise regarding the "do's" and "don'ts" after surgery. You and your family should read the instructions several times to familiarize yourselves thoroughly with them. Attempt to follow them faithfully, because those who do so generally have the smoothest post-operative course. This, of course, favors proper healing and a better result. Failure to follow these instructions faithfully can lead to certain complications which potentially could jeopardize the desired result. Whenever a question arises, refer back to this book. Chances are you will find the answer, but if you cannot please call us (832-956-1040). If you ever have a concern, call us. It is essential that our staff has the opportunity to evaluate any problem which may arise.

**Swelling**

Every operation, no matter how minor, is accompanied by swelling of the surrounding tissues. This is the body's way of helping the area heal. The amount of swelling varies from person to person, but it always seems more in the face because of its excellent blood supply. The increased blood supply to the region is responsible for the pink color of the skin and in some of the "discoloration" associated with surgery. The swelling becomes a little greater the second and third day after your operation, especially along the jaw line and around the eyes and ears. When this occurs, the face and neck feel tighter. Swelling is generally worse when you first arise in the morning (proof that it is better to stay up or elevated as much as possible). The swelling itself is not serious and is not an indication that something is going wrong with your healing. When these healing fluids are no longer required, the tissues release them and they are absorbed through the bloodstream.

You must be willing to accept temporary swelling, lumpiness, and discoloration which occur following such operations. Though usually visually disconcerting, most people feel it is a negligible inconvenience to pay for the physical and psychological improvement they generally experience.

If you feel the swelling is excessive, however, notify us so we can examine the areas in question. Many patients complain that one side of the face occasionally swells more than the other. This is to be expected.

The main thing to remember is that such swelling eventually subsides; you can help in several ways:

1. Stay up (sitting, standing, walking around) as much as possible after your first post-operative night. Of course, you should rest when you tire. It is important not to "push yourself" as you need your energy for your body to heal.
2. Avoid turning your head or bending at the neck. When you must turn, move the shoulders and head as one unit or as though you had a "stiff neck." Do this for two (2) weeks. Do not lie on the side of your face.
3. Avoid bending over or lifting heavy objects for one week. Besides aggravating swelling, this may raise the blood pressure and cause bleeding.
4. Avoid hitting or bumping your face and neck. It is wise not to pick up small children as their actions are often unpredictable, and you should sleep alone for two (2) weeks after your operation.
5. Sleep with the head of the bed elevated (or in a recliner) for 4-6 weeks after your operation. To accomplish this, place two or three pillows under the head of the mattress and one or two on top of it, but keep the back and neck in a straight line. Bend only at the waist. Try not to roll over on your face as this tends to tear down the supporting stitches used under

the skin of your face and may cause the scars behind the ears to widen. It is advisable to sleep on your back for two (2) weeks.

6. Avoid straining to go to the restroom. If you need a laxative, take one you are accustomed to using.

**Discoloration**

It is not unusual to have varying amounts of discoloration about the face. Like swelling, it may become more pronounced after the first day or so, but remember it is temporary. Most of it usually subsides within two (2) weeks, all the while decreasing in intensity. In some patients, especially those with thin, fair skin, the pink discoloration can last longer. This is a result of seeing the blood supply below the skin helping with the healing process.

You can camouflage discoloration (to some extent) by using a thicker makeup. A water-based makeup (two shades darker than your skin color) may be applied with a moist sponge; after it dries, a second layer may be applied. It can be removed with water. Do not apply makeup over the incisions themselves for several days after the sutures have been removed; however, you can bring it up close to the line of the incisions. Makeup should never be applied over any area of crusting as this increases the risk for infection.

**Turning the Head**

AVOID turning the head or stretching the neck. When you must turn, move the shoulders and head as one unit as though you had a "stiff neck." This should be performed for the first two (2) weeks. After this, you can begin to move your neck but do not pull against anything that feels tight or you can widen your scars.

**Discomfort**

The majority of patients have described little actual pain following a face lift, but for a while you may experience a tight sensation as a result of the swelling. This is very commonly felt behind the ears and below the chin. You may also get the sensation of your face feeling heavy as a result of the swelling. As is usually the case with such things, this seems worse later in the day, at night, and when one becomes nervous or worried.

If you should have any discomfort around the face, try the application of cold compresses (never ice or anything that comes directly out of the freezer) before resorting to prescription pain medication. The reason is that prescription pain relievers often cause sensations of light-headedness and nausea, particularly in the immediate post-operative period. They also cause constipation. As a result, they seem to make recovery more tedious. If cold compresses are not effective, you may first try the recommended over-the-counter pain medication. Under no circumstances should ASPIRIN, IBUPROFEN, NAPROXEN, or medications containing aspirin or salicylates be taken as this could increase your risk of bleeding and jeopardize your result. Be sure to check the labels of any pain medications you already have or any you purchase from the drug store. Medications with acetaminophen (Tylenol) do not increase bleeding but they should only be taken as directed. Your prescription pain medication will also have acetaminophen in it, and it is important to limit the total amount of acetaminophen you take in a day. Only take the medications as prescribed. If you have any questions, please ask us. If Tylenol® doesn't help your pain, then you should take the prescribed pain medication as directed.

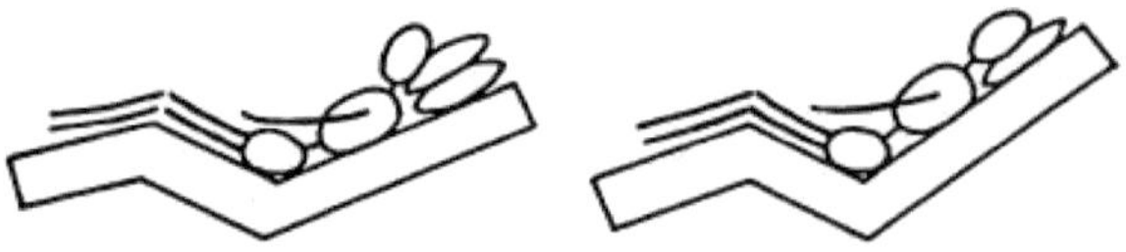


This demonstrates the appropriate sleeping position whereby the back and neck are in alignment. The improper position places undue strain on the back and neck causing pain.

When patients do complain of pain, the most common cause is improper posture while sleeping (see diagram above). The hips, back, and head should be in a straight line whenever one is lying down. Placing pillows to try to elevate your head will lead to an abnormal strain on the back and neck which may produce a spasm or "crick." These can be helped with massages, or treated with moist heat on the back of the neck and shoulders. Do not apply heat to the face or on the neck anywhere forward of the incision lines. In some circumstances, I may recommend an injection to help with the pain.

### Ice Compresses

Face towels (not an ice bag) dipped in a container of water and ice applied across the forehead, jaw, and neck several times daily during the first three (3) days may help reduce swelling, discomfort, and discoloration in the face. Continuing beyond this time is ok if you'd like although it likely will not decrease the swelling any faster. It is important to not overdo the cold compresses as they can irritate your skin. The facial garment worn the first day after surgery can be used to help secure the cold compresses in place for your convenience.

### Removal of Dressings

An elastic pressure dressing will be applied before you leave the operating room. This is designed to help the healing process. The dressing is to remain in place until the following morning. You should be as quiet as possible during this time to help the healing; therefore, a great deal of talking and having too many visitors are discouraged. If your dressing becomes too uncomfortable, report it to us, but do not remove or loosen it without our direction. Failure to follow this can negatively affect your final result.

### Elevate the Head of Bed

To help minimize swelling, it is recommended that you sleep on your back in a recliner elevated at 30-40 degrees for a minimum of two (2) weeks. Continuing to sleep elevated for 6 weeks will help the remaining swelling disappear more quickly if you are able to tolerate it. If you are unable to sleep in a recliner your bed can be utilized with the head of the bed elevated 30-40 degrees. Remember to keep the back and neck in a straight line instead of just propping up your neck on pillows as this would only lead to a stiff neck. You will notice that if you lay flat at night then when you awake in the morning your swelling will be greater and take longer to go away.

### Getting Out of Bed

We usually recommend that you remain in bed but with the head of your bed elevated during the first twelve (12) hours following surgery. When you get up to go to the bathroom make sure that someone has a hold of you to guide you. After the first 12 hours, you may sit in a chair or walk around your room with someone holding you. You will notice about 24-48 hours after surgery you should be able to do these activities without assistance, although having someone around will make it easier for you.

### Hemorrhage

It is normal to have a small amount of blood on your bandages and dressings. If bleeding is continuous lay down, elevate the head, and apply ice compresses and steady pressure about that area of face and neck. Notify the Clinic by telephone (832-956-1040) for any bleeding that is not stopping with conservative measures or if you are concerned.

### Temperature

Generally, the body temperature rises close to 100 degrees following a face lift as a result to the healing process. Patients will often think they have an increased temperature because they feel warm. It is more common in the later afternoon to feel this way as the body is naturally warmer in the afternoon and colder around 3 AM. If you feel warm you should measure your temperature by mouth. Report any persistent temperature above 100 degrees, measured at least twice and two (2) hours apart, as it could be an early sign of an infection.

### Weakness

After a person has an anesthetic or has undergone any type of operation, they may feel weak, break out in "cold sweats," or get dizzy. This is a normal reaction and gradually clears up in a few days without medication.

Insomnia

You will be prescribed a sleeping medication. It is recommended you take one the night before surgery to help you get a good night's rest. After surgery, if you have difficulty sleeping you may continue to use the sleep aid as prescribed. It should be remembered that such drugs also tend to make some people feel light-headed or weak and should be taken only if needed. For those patients who do not like prescription sleep aids then two (2) Tylenol ® PM may be of benefit. It is important not to have more Tylenol ® (acetaminophen) than recommended in a 24-hour period as it can lead to liver failure. Keep in mind that any prescribed pain medication also has acetaminophen and needs to be accounted for.

### Depression

Leading up to surgery it is normal to be anxious, excited, nervous, etc. Once the surgery occurs, it is not unusual for an individual to go through a brief period of depression. No matter how much they wanted the operation beforehand and how much they were informed about what to expect postoperatively, patients are concerned when they see their face swollen and bruised. This occurs in almost 50% of patients to some degree.

Be patient and realize that this is a temporary condition which will subside shortly. The best "treatment" consists of busying one's self with the details of post-operative care and trying to divert one's attention to other thoughts (T.V., a book, an unhurried walk in a peaceful place).

### Numbness

Parts of the face, neck, ears, and scalp sometimes feel numb after the face lift operation. This is to be expected and is usually temporary. It may take several weeks or, on rare occasions, months for this to subside. As the feeling returns you will note "pings and zings" as well as itching which represents the nerves growing back. The top of the head may itch or exhibit numbness for 6-12 months in some cases. It is important not to itch these areas when you are numb. It is better to use a single finger and place it on the area that is itching. This will prevent you from harming yourself by rubbing too hard which could lead to hair loss.

### Tightness of the Face

The skin of the face may feel tight for a while and you may feel that it interferes with normal facial expressions. As the swelling goes down this should disappear within a few weeks.

### Thinning of the Hair

There may be thinning of the hair in areas adjacent to the suture lines in the temple, forehead, scalp, and behind the ears. This happens less than 10% of the time. If it does appear, it tends to happen about 3 months after the surgery. This can sometimes be avoided by closely adhering to the instructions about shampooing and cleaning the suture lines. Should a problem arise, we will advise you on any additional recommended treatments although the problem tends to resolve on its own.

### If You Injure Your Face

Many individuals sustain accidental hits on the face during the early post-operative period. You need not be concerned unless the blow is hard or if bleeding or considerable swelling ensues. Call us immediately (832-956-1040) if you are concerned, or report the incident at the next Clinic visit.

### Your Medications

When discharged after surgery you will be given instructions concerning the medicines you were prescribed prior to surgery. Take these as directed. In most cases these prescriptions need not be refilled. The antibiotic may on occasion cause an upset stomach or diarrhea. If this occurs, please inform us so the medication may be changed. Do not stop an antibiotic without informing us.

### Resuming Activities

1. WEARING GLASSES AND CONTACT LENSES: Eyeglasses may be worn as soon as the bandages are removed. It is important to have the sides of the glasses higher than normal so they do not rest or rub against your suture line. Contact lenses may be inserted the day after surgery, unless you have had eyelid surgery at which point you need to wait ten (10) days.
2. HAIR AND BODY CARE: You may wash your hair with lukewarm water in a shower and carefully comb it out with a large toothed-comb the day after surgery. Do not use hot water. You may use shampoo and take a shower beginning on the second postoperative day, but NEVER on the day you have had sutures and clips removed. Hair coloring and permanents should also be delayed until six (6) weeks after your surgery.
    A. Do not tweeze the eyebrows for one week.
3. HOUSEHOLD ACTIVITIES: For the first two (2) weeks do not perform any activities that require you to bend over, elevate your heart rate, or elevate your body temperature as this could stimulate bleeding. After this time, you may slowly reintroduce your daily household activities as tolerated but listen to your body and do not strain yourself.
4. PULL-OVER CLOTHING: During the first two weeks, you should wear clothing that fastens either in the front or the back rather than the type that must be pulled over the head. This is to prevent you from pulling open your incisions.

5. ATHLETICS: No swimming, strenuous athletic activity, or exercises that involve turning the head for four (4) weeks. Walking is recommended after two (2) weeks. Jogging should be delayed until four (4) weeks.
6. KEEPING A "STIFF" FACE AND NECK: You should not move the face and neck excessively until the skin heals to the underlying tissues.
7. AVOID anything that feels uncomfortable.
8. DON'T TURN THE HEAD without turning the neck and shoulders as one unit for the first two (2) weeks.
9. DON'T BEND the head forward or extend the neck backward for the same period.
10. AVOID gum or foods that are hard to chew as you will notice this would cause a pain in front of your ear. Soft foods and soups are recommended to minimize this possibility of pain for two (2) weeks.
11. AVOID yawning with the mouth opened widely for two (2) weeks.
12. RETURNING TO WORK AND RESUMING SOCIAL ACTIVITIES: When you should return to work depends on the amount of physical activity and also the amount of swelling and discoloration you develop. The average patient may return to work or go out socially approximately two (2) weeks after surgery. At this point you will still be a little swollen but most patients would still appear better than preoperatively. Individual responses to surgery vary with the number of simultaneous procedures, age, and general well-being of the patient, so the actual return date will depend on a number of factors. If your neck was lifted, do not drive for two (2) weeks. If it wasn't lifted then once you are no longer taking pain medication you should be able to drive if you feel up to it.

### Your Scars

After all stitches and clips have been removed, the scars will appear deep pink in color. This represents the increased blood flow to the area to promote healing. There will be varying amounts of swelling in and around the scars themselves. With the passage of time, the pink should become white, the firmness of the scar should soften, and they should become less noticeable. But if you stretch them, expect them to respond by getting thicker in order to "protect" themselves.

Some crusting may occur around incision sites. Cleaning the incisions as directed followed by applying the recommended ointment can soften these crusts and improve the healing process.

Each individual varies with respect to healing, but it takes approximately one year before the scar turns to a fine white line and the healing process finishes. Should you not be healing as well as we would like, other measures can be taken to improve scarring. This is why it is important to follow up as scheduled. However, scars are usually easily camouflaged by makeup and hairstyling

### Follow-up Clinic Visits

Before leaving for home, you should check with the secretary at the Clinic for an appointment. This should be done soon because special preparations must be made for this visit in advance of your arrival as these are different from the pre-operative routine.

Don't build up a feeling of fear and anxiety about post-operative visits. A few of the skin sutures may be removed and the progress of your healing will be checked. Removing sutures is quick and uncomplicated because it is done with small delicate instruments to minimize discomfort. Sutures that aren't blue dissolve by themselves but sometimes are removed to speed up healing at the same times as your blue sutures. You will probably feel much better after your Clinic visit. Ordinarily, ALL SUTURES and CLIPS are removed within one week from the day of your surgery. The exception is a little blue suture at the bottom of each ear which remains in place for two (2) weeks. During this interim, do not disturb the sutures or clips yourself. Crusting will occur around the sutures which is why the daily cleaning instructions are recommended. We will soften and remove some of the crusts during each Clinic visit as well to promote healing.

**Post-Operative Instructions**

1. For the incisions around the front and back of the ears use hydrogen peroxide on a Q-tip or cotton ball to clean your incisions six (6) times daily. Apply the recommended antibiotic ointment in the same locations you used the hydrogen peroxide. Do not apply the ointment to areas that have hair on both sides of the incision such as in the scalp as the ointment will not get to the incisions and you will make a mess of your hair.
2. The next day after surgery let warm water run through the hair while standing in a shower. Two (2) days after surgery you may use a recommended shampoo. If you had eyelid surgery do not be afraid to get the sutures around eyes wet when showering. You should shampoo at least daily for the first postoperative week. Never rub any of your wounds with the towel. Pat the areas dry.
3. Report any of the warning signs of infection such as sudden or excessive localized swelling, redness, drainage, fever, or worsening pain.
4. Avoid taking medications on an empty stomach as they may produce nausea. This is especially true for any prescribed pain medications. Some medications, especially antibiotics, can produce digestive system upset such as diarrhea or nausea. If this occurs, please notify us so we can change the antibiotic and prescribe any nausea pills if needed
5. Never wash your hair the day that sutures, clips or staples are removed. Wash it the following day.
6. Hair sprays, conditioners and vegetable color rinses (Roux®) can be used in two weeks if resurfacing procedures were not performed.
7. Make sure you keep all post-operative appointments as the instructions may change based on how your body is healing.
8. Avoid excessive sunning of the face for one (1) month; ordinary exposure is not harmful but if your scars get a "tan" they may always be darker than the surrounding skin.
9. Avoid smoking or very smoky areas for two weeks. Nicotine, whether inhaled, ingested, chewed, "vaped," or absorbed from patches, may result in delayed wound healing and increased scarring. Having nicotine in your blood at the time of surgery increases your risk of having problems by a factor of 17.

**WEEK 1**

(Beginning the day after surgery)

DO: Clean suture lines located around the front and back of the ear with hydrogen peroxide on a Q-tip or cotton ball 6 times daily, decreasing the frequency as instructed.

DO: Apply the recommended antibiotic ointment to the suture lines following cleaning.

DO: Shower on the first postoperative day (once). Allow warm water, without soap or shampoo, to run though the hair. Some hair and possibly old blood will be noted in the rinse at this time.

DO: Shower once daily starting on the second post-operative day. Clean the scalp with the recommended shampoo only. Continue the showers once daily for one week. If you had a skin resurfacing procedure, try to keep water and shampoo away from the resurfaced areas.

DO: Clean your face while in the shower gently with soap taking care to clean in an upward direction just as your lift was performed.

DO: Elevate the head of the bed 30 to 40 degrees for 4-6 weeks (at least 2) to help minimize swelling but keep the back and neck in a straight line to prevent discomfort. Sleeping in a recliner can make this easier and more comfortable.

DO: Apply facial cold compresses several times daily for the first three days to reduce swelling and discomfort. After this time, cold compresses likely will not improve any swelling or discoloration but can still feel nice if you'd like to continue them.

DO: Wash your face with lukewarm water.

DO: Wear eyeglasses, if necessary, keeping them off of your incisions.

DO: Wear contacts, if necessary, unless eyelid surgery was also performed. If eyelid surgery was performed wait 10 days before inserting your contacts.

* * * * *

DO NOT: Pull your ear forward while cleaning behind the ear as this can stimulate bleeding and lead to a worse scar.

DO NOT: Use any hair sprays or conditioners for the first 2 weeks. Do not use hair coloring or get a permanent for 6 weeks.

DO NOT: Apply makeup to the face for the first week and do not apply makeup to the incision lines until instructed to do so.

DO NOT: Use a curling iron for 4 weeks.

MEN: Do not shave for the first week. Electric razors are recommended for the first six (6) weeks.

**WEEK 2**

DO: Wash your face with a mild soap twice daily using only your finger-tips and not a cloth. Avoid washing resurfaced areas until instructed.

DO: Continue cleaning and wound care as described above, especially if crusts along incisions are still present. This is usually continued for 2-3 days after your sutures and clips are removed.

DO: Start applying powder-based makeup to your face except areas of continued crusting. Do not use makeup on resurfaced areas until instructed

MEN: Shave with an electric razor only. Do not use a straight razor as this is more likely to cause small cuts which could lead to infections.

**WEEK 3**

DO: Restart Retin-A use at this time if applicable, but not over resurfaced areas.

DO: Use an SPF 30 sunscreen over healed incisions if sun exposure is expected, but not over resurfaced areas. If healing incisions get a tan, they will always be darker than the surrounding skin.

DO: Resume regular physical activity but ease into your activity and listen to your body.

**WEEK 5**

DO: Use oil-based makeup if desired.

DO: Start using a curling iron. Be careful not to injure areas of the scalp that may still be numb.

**WEEK 7**

DO: Color hair and obtain a permanent if desired.

**Remember the things you were told before your operation, namely:**

1. When the bandages are first removed, the face will appear swollen and there will be varying amounts of discoloration and lumpiness. These conditions will subside to a very large extent within two (2) weeks; however, it will take 6-8 weeks for ninety (90) % of the swelling to disappear and for your face to reach a natural contour. With make-up and hair styling most patients can go out after two (2) weeks without any great concern. Most face lift patients look their very best at about 3-4 months after surgery.
2. Any discoloration will gradually disappear over a period of 10-14 days in most cases.
3. Swelling and lumpiness persists in front of the ears and below the chin a while longer than other regions. For those with little facial fat, you may even be able to feel the deep sutures initially but they are absorbable. This will improve with time.
4. A tight feeling behind and below the ears is to be expected for a few weeks after surgery. Do not pull against this.
5. If you had any skin resurfacing procedure in conjunction with your face lift, please follow the instructions for post-operative care for those regions. Failure to comply may result in delayed healing and scarring.
6. Most of all, BE PATIENT during the healing process. It truly is a process. If you have further questions, you are urged to call us and keep your appointments.

**Report to The Clinic Any:**

1. Temperature elevation greater than 100 degrees
2. Sudden swelling or discoloration.
3. Hemorrhage.
4. Discharge from the wound edges or other evidence of infection.
5. Development of any reaction to medications.

If you have any questions call

832-956-1040

# Chapter 12

## Skin Rejuvenation

**The Skin as an Organ**

**Advanced Skin Rejuvenation**

**Treatment for Wrinkles**

**Laser Resurfacing**

*The Right Laser for the Right Conditions*
*The Laser Treatment*

**Chemical Peeling**

*Limitations and Restrictions*
*Pertinent Facts You Should Know*
*Chemical Peeling: Stages of Healing*

**Dermabrasion**

*The Treatment*
*After Dermabrasion*

**After Facial Skin Resurfacing**

*Swelling*
*Discomfort*
*Skin Appearance*
*"Fever Blisters"*
*Medications*
*Depression*
*Resuming Activities*
*Postoperative Clinic Visits and Accommodations*
*Post-Operative Instructions*
*Remember the things you were told before your operation, namely*
*Report to the Clinic Any*

## The Skin as an Organ

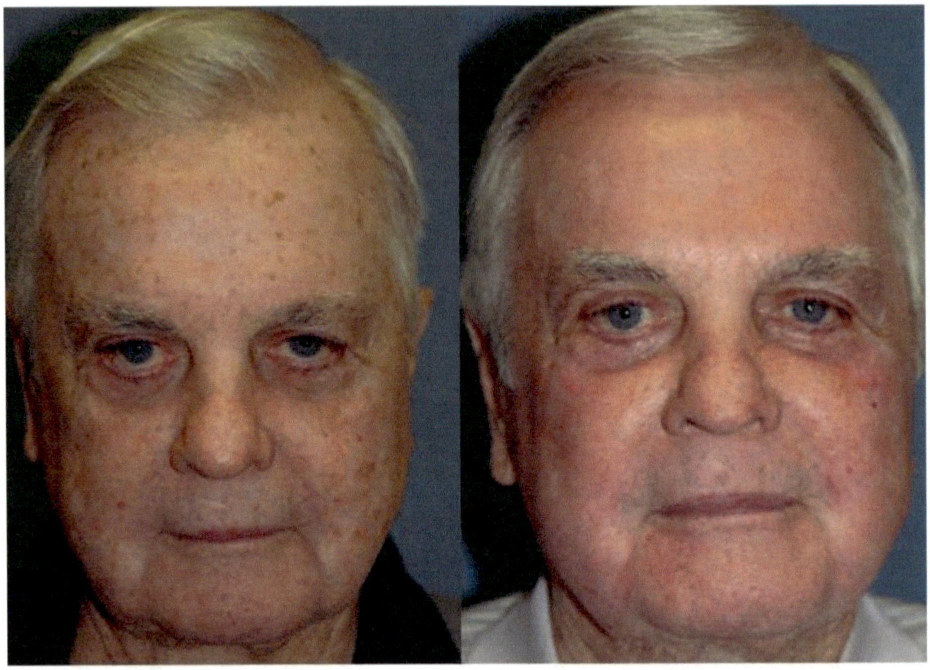

Before After

This patient is 10 days out after receiving a Baker's solution full face chemical peel. He had a history of multiple precancerous skin lesions removed. Skin resurfacing can help to prevent these types of lesions from becoming a real cancer. You can notice the overall improvement in the quality and texture of his skin. You can also see the improvement in his age spots (most are now gone). His skin still has a pink tone which is common this soon after any skin resurfacing but this should resolve with time. Although he received his resurfacing to help to prevent skin cancers, skin resurfacing is more commonly done as a way to improve the skin quality and fine wrinkles.

Most people do not realize this, but the skin is the largest organ of the human body. It serves many important functions including protection from the environment, heat regulation, and preventing damage from UV light. Despite its important function, the skin is often neglected until the signs of aging are already present.

The damaging effects of the sun to the skin cannot be overstated. It can lead to premature aging, sun spots, and even skin cancers. As you age you will notice a change in the overall quality and texture of your skin. Fine wrinkles begin to develop. The outer layer of skin may thicken and become rougher whereas the deeper layers lose elasticity and begin to droop. Sun damage leads to pigment (color changes) and even early skin cancers. A complete facial rejuvenation involves addressing the skin.

## Advanced Skin Rejuvenation

Some surgeons and aestheticians refer to the procedures herein described as a "non-surgical face lift." Although small amounts of skin tightening do occur, to refer to them as a face lift is misleading. They are quite helpful to improve the quality and appearance of the skin, but they are used to treat different signs of aging than a face lift treats. Superficial layers of skin can be removed by a variety of methods of skin resurfacing including chemical peeling, dermabrasion, and laser resurfacing. Each method has unique qualities and an experienced surgeon can explain which procedure(s) might be the most advantageous in your case.

With any of these methods, outer layers of the sun damaged, wrinkled, or scarred skin are removed. The treatments can be superficial, intermediate, or deep. However, only with the intermediate and deeper procedures are new collagen and elastic fibers produced. As a result, some tightening of facial tissues occurs, but not to the extent which can be accomplished with surgical removal through conventional face lifting and eyelid lifting techniques.

Superficial peels generally do not produce long-term improvement in the quality and texture of the skin, but may be used as adjuncts to the methods herein described. They are beneficial from the standpoint that they have the least downtime and can be repeated frequently. They are best characterized as skin polishers as they will improve the skin temporarily. This can prove useful for those with minimal skin damage who have an event coming up in the following weeks and cannot have the downtime seen with deeper resurfacing techniques.

## Treatment for Wrinkles

A face lift, eyelid surgery (blepharoplasty), or a brow lift cannot successfully remove the wrinkles of weather-beaten skin, the transverse creases of the forehead, "crow's feet" around the eyes nor the vertical wrinkles of the upper and lower lips completely. They will provide some benefit to these areas by taking out the "slack" in the skin but the etched-on wrinkles in the skin will still remain. Remember, surgery is designed to improve sags, bags, and bulges seen at rest and resurfacing should improve wrinkles present at rest. Botox or another neuromodulator helps to improve the conditions present with activity. Depending on your skin condition, amount of downtime you can afford, and your desired result, dermabrasion, chemical peeling, and/or laser resurfacing may be recommended. But every person's skin is different, and we will recommend which combination of procedures might be best for your skin.

Skin resurfacing may be done as an isolated procedure (for example around the lips, around the eyes, or the entire face) or it may be used as an adjunct to face lifting and eyelid surgery in an overall facial rejuvenation program. Certain areas can be resurfaced at the same time as a facelift, but I recommend waiting at least a few days following surgery to consider a full-face resurfacing to ensure that your skin is healing well from surgery. Performing a face lift and full-face resurfacing at the same time can sometimes be too much for you skin to heal although there are some exceptions to this.

Some skin types are more favorable than others; fair complexions tend to do better than darker ones. Thick, tough, more deeply etched, or oily skins may require a two-staged approach for the best results (i.e., a second peel or "touch up" of several areas at a later time). Like painting a roughly textured wall, deep creases may require a "touch-up."

Resurfacing can sometimes produce a dramatic improvement in the texture of the skin of your face. It may be the best treatment available to the facial plastic surgeon to help obtain a fresher, more youthful skin. Certainly, it is not indicated for every patient; therefore, we will give you our opinion as to whether we feel you are a candidate for these procedures. Resurfacing alone is not indicated for treatment of sagging tissues. Although the new skin has better elasticity, sagging requires surgery.

Skin resurfacing is considered a surgical procedure, therefore the risks that apply to surgery must be considered. Patients are warned that taking female hormones or birth control pills for approximately six months after a resurfacing may have a higher chance of the skin darkening temporarily. This can usually be remedied with a topical cream if it were to happen. Patients who feel they must take hormones usually do so without incurring any problems, but the risk of a darker skin exists.

Some degree of swelling follows any surgical procedure. The swelling is due to the new tissue fluids brought into the area by the body to promote healing. The increased blood supply to the region is responsible for the pink color of the skin and is some of the "discoloration" associated with surgery, particularly with chemical peeling. When these healing fluids are no longer required, the tissues release them and they are absorbed through the bloodstream.

One must be willing to accept the swelling and discoloration which occurs following such operations. Though swelling itself is usually visually disconcerting most people feel it is a negligible inconvenience to pay for the physical and psychological improvement they generally experience. **Please inform us if you have taken Accutane** as you cannot have any resurfacing procedure for at least 1 year following its use to prevent scarring.

Post-operative care is extremely important in your obtaining the best result. This is more so following skin resurfacing than any other procedure in this book. We will give you instructions to assist you in caring for your new skin. Your "new skin" will be much like the skin of a newborn baby in that it will take time for it to toughen and be able to tolerate direct sun, wind exposure, and certain skin care products. Because it is "new" skin the texture and color will be somewhat different from that which has not been resurfaced. Makeup can generally camouflage any contrast and Dr. Guy blends the resurfacing treatments at the edges to help minimize this as well. Continued care of your new skin is important to help maintain what has been done with resurfacing. A good skin care program is recommended and we have several options available through our Clinic.

# Laser Resurfacing

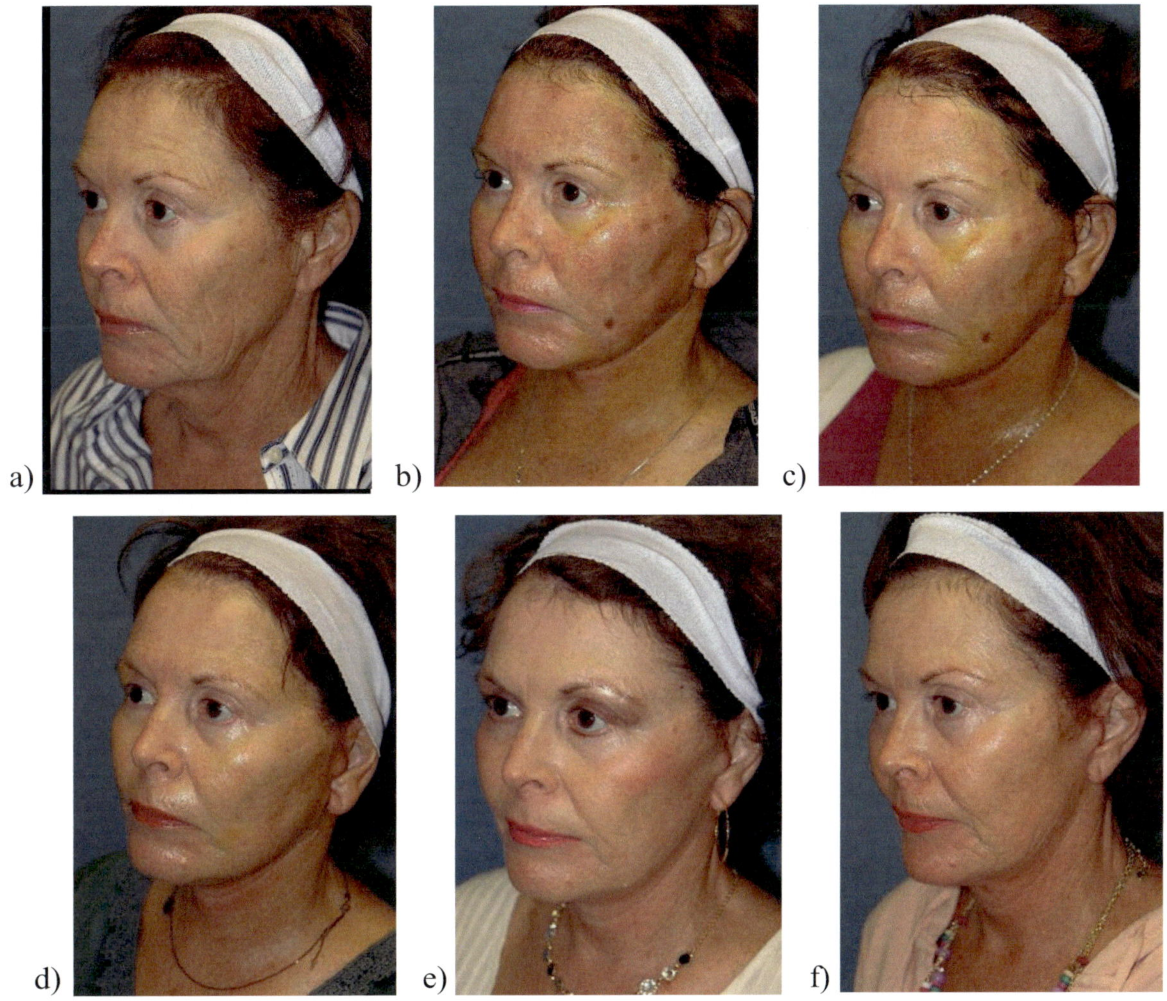


a) Day 0 b) Day 1 c) Day 2 d) Day 8 e) Day 19 f) Day 120

This patient underwent a facelift followed by a full-face laser resurfacing procedure. Notice her progression of healing and discoloration. By 8 days most of her discoloration is gone and the brown spots present before treatment are nearly gone. By day 19 she was back wearing makeup. By day 120 he results from her resurfacing continued to last showing the improvements are not a result of swelling but actually from the development of the new, healthier skin.

### The Right Laser for the Right Conditions

There are hundreds of different types of lasers and machines for light therapy. Each one does something slightly different than the other. Others use the same laser but are manufactured by a different company which creates a unique marketing name. Many are marketed using an older technology with a new name and a slight tweak to the laser.

Although there are many similarities amongst lasers, all are not the same. They come in a variety of different forms, and are designed to perform different tasks. Some lasers vaporize the outer layers of sun damaged or aging skin ($CO_2$, fractionated $CO_2$, Erbium:YAG). Some can also pass through the outer layers of the skin and destroy deeper birthmarks such as port wine stains, tiny blood vessels, and Rosacea (pulse dyed laser). Various lasers and light therapy can help in the reduction of unanted hair. In addition, IPL or the photo facial can help improve sun spots, veins, red spots, and skin quality with several treatments.

As is the case with most technology, there is an art to doing it. In order to obtain the maximum benefit, experience is required. Lasers, like any technology, must be used for the right reasons. The right reason is that a particular technology is superior to other forms of treatment. For some conditions, lasers exceed other forms of treatment. We offer several different resurfacing lasers and IPL to help customize a treatment for your skin.

### The Laser Treatment

Laser therapy can be performed in the clinic with the use of topical and local anesthetics combined with oral pills. This is what most patients elect to undergo as there is a significant cost saving. However, there can still be some discomfort associated with this so some patients elect to undergo the treatment in a local surgical center with the use of an anesthesiologist or nurse anesthetist to provide a greater degree of comfort. For these patients, a full-face chemical peel will be used instead as the laser is not able to be transported. It should be noted this latter option does add a significant amount to the cost if the procedure is performed in isolation. Depending on the areas being treated, laser resurfacing can take up to an hour for a full-face therapy. For isolated treatment areas, the timing is much less.

## Chemical Peeling

A "chemical peel" involves the careful application of a scientifically formulated solution to the skin which later causes the top layer to separate and shed (like a blister) taking with it the sun-damaged and wrinkled layers. Swelling of the peeled area may be pronounced for the first few days but subsides dramatically after 5-7 days.

As mentioned previously, peels can be performed to a superficial, medium or deep depth. With medium and deep peels, it is much like having a sunburn or a blister in that the top layer of skin begins to "peel off" over a 4-5-day period revealing the fresh new skin underneath. Powder makeup may be used approximately one week after a superficial peel, two weeks after a medium depth peel, and three weeks after the application of a deep peel. These are all averages and may differ for you. Most patients may return to work or go out socially at these times. When instructions and precautions are heeded by the patient, the redness of the skin slowly subsides with the deeper the peel the longer it takes for the pink to go away. In most patients, this occurs within 6 to 8 weeks for deeper peels and within the week for superficial peels. For medium depth peels it takes approximately 4 weeks.

## Limitations and Restrictions

Avoidance of prolonged exposure to sunlight (as in sun bathing, golfing, tennis, etc.) is the biggest limitation. For deep depth peels this may be for up to three (3) to six (6) months because the "new" skin must build up a tolerance to the elements. Failure to follow this very important rule can cause some patients to develop pigmentation issues and skin irritation. For superficial peels this is limited usually to the first week. For medium depth peels depending on your skin type it can last up to a few months but is usually only restricted for the first month. With the judicious use of sun screen products and large brimmed hats these restrictions can sometimes be loosened. Ask about any activity you question prior to undergoing any resurfacing procedure as the post peel care of your skin is paramount to achieve the desired result.

Neither surgery nor resurfacing can correct wrinkles that occur only during facial expressions. The creases around the eyes produced by smiling, the forehead creases that occur with frowning, and the vertical lines in the upper lip that occur with puckering the lips for the most part are due to the contraction of the muscles of facial expression. None of the surgical procedures discussed in this book are able to eliminate the preceding conditions. If wrinkles and creases are present at rest then resurfacing combined with surgery may improve them. For those wrinkles only present with activity, Botox or a similar neuromodulator may be of benefit.

In our experience, the results have generally been very good. The degree of improvement for a surgical skin peel is transient, lasting for a period of time measured in years for the medium and deeper peels.

## Pertinent Facts You Should Know

1. With medium and deep chemical peeling, the solution stings as it is applied, but this is short-lived. Later discomfort can be eased with appropriate medications.
2. Considerable swelling may occur for a few days. The deeper the peel the greater the amount of swelling. The patient must be emotionally mature enough and be willing to accept this temporary distortion of appearance in order to achieve the desired end result. It is best to warn family members about this beforehand to avoid any surprises and unwarranted/ unwanted reactions.
3. The procedure may be performed in our clinic or in one of the local outpatient surgical facilities depending on the recommended peel.
4. When instructions are followed by patients, scarring following peeling is extremely rare. Failure to follow instructions can allow the controlled peel to extend deeper which is the cause of scarring
5. Deeper red areas that develop after a week may be treated with topical steroids.
6. Should red lumpy areas occur, they are softened with steroid injections. Several treatments might be required.
7. You should read the postoperative instructions prior to your consultation and treatment to ensure you are willing to accept the required downtime and postoperative care.

**Chemical Peeling: Stages of Healing**

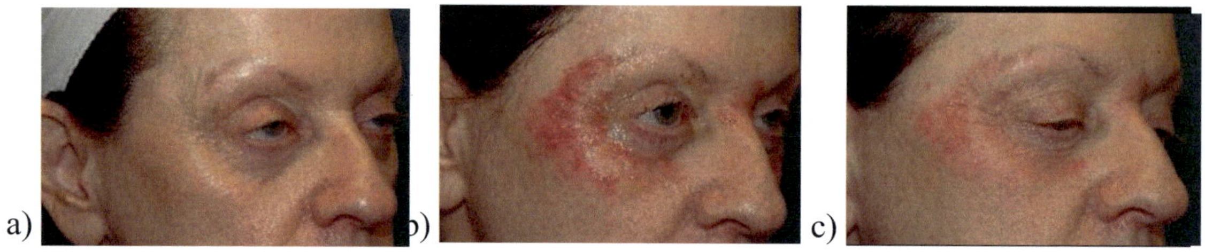

a) Day 0 b) Day 5 c) Day 8

This patient underwent a deep Baker-Gordon phenol peel to improve the static wrinkles around her eyes. You can see the progression in the appearance from the bright red and flaky tissue to the light pink seen at day 8. This pink slowly faded over the course of the subsequent weeks.

## Dermabrasion

When the skin has an irregular or uneven texture from acne scarring or from previous injuries/scars, dermabrasion may be the most effective. The technique of dermabrasion is similar to sanding a scratch from a wooden table in that the work is actually done on the elevated areas in an attempt to take them down closer to the level of the defect. When successful, this diminishes the crevices which are responsible for casting shadows when light strikes the face from an angle. The end result is skin that is somewhat smoother and tighter than before. When the texture of the skin is very irregular from excessive or deep scarring, a second treatment may be required 6-12 months after the initial treatment. This is because there is a limitation of how deep the original treatment can go. As the tissue heals and the new layer of skin forms, a second treatment may be performed.

The more superficial defects might be completely removed by dermabrasion. Those which are moderately deep may be improved but not removed and some of the deeper or "icepick" type scars may not be improved at all. Ice pick acne scars are often best treated by surgically removing them and then dermabrading the resulting scar. Prior to surgery it is difficult to predict the degree of improvement, and each patient's skin responds to the same treatment by the same surgeon in a different manner.

When dermabrasion is done as a part of a treatment for scar revision, it can provide the finishing touch to help smooth the tissues after the initial procedures have been completed. In some cases, only dermabrasion may be required for scars resulting from accidents. The degree of improvement will be determined in part by the severity of the condition treated. **Please inform us if you have taken Accutane for acne as resurfacing cannot be performed for at least one year after your last Accutane treatment to minimize the risk of scarring.**

### The Treatment

Dermabrasion is usually performed at the office for minor procedures. For larger treatment areas and full-face treatment, it is performed at one of the local surgical centers under "Twilight Anesthesia" and local anesthesia. The surgery is relatively painless since the skin is anesthetized during the procedure. There can be minor stinging for the remainder of the day and this usually responds to over-the-counter pain medication. With the techniques we use, pain is rarely a problem. Since dermabrasion is a surgical procedure, the risks of the surgery should be considered and understood prior to proceeding.

### After Dermabrasion

As is the case with all resurfacing treatments, the final result will not be apparent immediately after dermabrasion. During the healing period the face demonstrates a deep pink or red color which should fade dramatically within a week or two. In some cases, several months may pass before the healing is completed.

For most patients within about 2-3 weeks, makeup may be worn to cover any residual discoloration and patients may return to work, school, or resume their normal indoor social activities. To prevent skin irritation and prolonged redness, do not use makeup until directed to do so by Dr. Guy. And since the skin of the treated area will be "new" skin, it will need to be cared for as one would care for a new baby's skin. Just as you would not put a newborn in the sun for an extended period, direct sunlight during the early stages of healing is discouraged. As with any resurfacing, this can irritate the skin, lead to extended redness, and lead to color changes of the skin especially without the judicious use of sunscreen products. Since the treated area will possess "new" skin it is understandable that the skin tones and texture may vary from the untreated areas. I employ techniques to minimize this at the time of your treatment to help blend the area with the surrounding untreated areas. Proper makeup application at the appropriate time should further camouflage this condition.

## After Facial Skin Resurfacing

The following instructions are designed to answer practically every question regarding the "Do's" and "Don'ts" following these procedures. You and your family should read these instructions several times and become thoroughly familiar with them. Faithful adherence to these instructions tends to result in the smoothest post-operative course and most favorable healing. Whenever a question arises, refer back to this section; more than likely you will find the answer. If you still are unsure, by all means, telephone the Clinic (832-956-1040).

Failure to follow these instructions faithfully can lead to certain complications which potentially could jeopardize the desired result and lead to scarring.

### Swelling

As you were informed before surgery, you can expect moderate to severe swelling in the areas treated, especially around the eyes and lips. Unlike other procedures where cold compresses can be used to minimize the swelling, they cannot be used on resurfaced skin as they can irritate the skin. Remember this is only temporary. Swelling reaches its peak by the second or third day and should begin to subside by the fourth or fifth day. You can help decrease the amount of swelling by keeping your head elevated about 30 to 40 degrees when reclining and by staying up (sitting, standing, walking around) as much as possible. Sometimes the medications which are prescribed may help reduce the swelling, but gravity and time are more reliable.

### Discomfort

Following the application of the peel solution, there is a stinging pain which lasts for a few seconds. The stinging quickly disappears but returns within several minutes. When it returns it persists for six (6) to eight (8) hours, occasionally longer. This type of discomfort can usually be relieved by taking the prescribed pain tablets. In addition, I inject a longer acting local anesthesia to help keep the face numb during this time period.

For lasers and dermabrasion, it creates the sensation of a mild sunburn for the first evening. This is also improved in the same manner as a chemical peel.

After the first night, discomfort should be negligible and can usually be relieved by aspirin. In fact, aspirin is the medication of choice for the pain associated with this type of procedure **if this is the only procedure you underwent**. If you have undergone any other procedures at the same time then you CANNOT use aspirin as it would increase your risk of bleeding. If you are unsure then use Tylenol or the prescribed pain medication.

### Skin Appearance

Immediately after a chemical peel the skin will have a brownish hue. Following a laser treatment, the skin has tiny red spots in a grid like pattern. After dermabrasion, the skin is very red similar to what you see with a rug burn and produces an amber color fluid. Within twenty-four (24) to thirty-six (36) hours the treated areas resemble a deep sunburn, blister, or abrasion, and you may notice an amber fluid oozing from the skin. This is expected because the superficial layers of skin have been removed from the deeper layer.

During the first week, you will notice the skin will crust and begin flaking. With the topical ointments, these crusts will soften. Beginning around the 3$^{rd}$ to 7$^{th}$ day the crusts will begin to flake off with most of the crusts gone by the 10$^{th}$ day. For those who faithfully apply their ointments, you may never see any crusts. The lower lid region is usually the last area in which crusting disappears. Never pick at crusts or pieces of skin that do not loosen easily. Picking off one of these crusts could lead to bleeding and scarring. Crusting sheds naturally with time and topical treatment. Apply the recommended topical dressing and try to leave it in place until instructed otherwise. As the ointments are not formulated for the eyes, avoid getting softening agents in your eyes as this can irritate them. Once the crusts have fallen off the new skin will appear intensely pink.

The intense pink color usually fades rapidly after the second week but some pink color will remain for up to six (6) to eight (8) weeks, continually decreasing in intensity. For a while, the skin usually appears somewhat tense and slightly scaly. The finer wrinkles and the deep grooves, however, should also be less evident.

Try to keep the fingers, facial tissues, cotton balls or Q-tips away from the face. Fingertips contain bacteria and oils and have been in contact with soaps, nail care products and other materials which might irritate the delicate new skin. Facial tissues and cotton can leave behind irritating fibers. Do not wear a shower cap or head band that comes in contact with any area which has been resurfaced. This might result in delayed healing and jeopardize an otherwise good result.

Within about 2-3 weeks many patients can use makeup over the resurfaced areas but only once cleared by myself. If you begin wearing makeup too soon it can prolong the healing process. Mineral powder based makeup will be recommended initially with oil based makeup delayed for several weeks.

Occasionally small "white cysts" may appear in the treated areas. They are stopped-up oil glands and usually disappear in two (2) to three (3) weeks without specific treatment. If they persist, we can demonstrate a technique to help eliminate them.

Early in the healing process, exposure to heat, cold, wind or emotional upset (fear, anger, crying, etc.) will cause the skin to temporarily become intensely pink. This is due to increased blood flow or "blushing." After about three (3) to four (4) months, this phenomenon should disappear. Each time we have witnessed prolonged redness or irritation of resurfaced skin, we have found that something in the patient's environment and/or self-administered skin care treatments contribute to the problem.

### "Fever Blisters"

Patients who have had difficulty with recurrent "fever blisters" or "cold sores" may develop an exacerbation of these lesions four (4) or five (5) days post-operatively. All patients undergoing resurfacing around the mouth will be prescribed an antiviral medication to help prevent them from developing. It is important to take this as directed. If you do notice the sensation of a fever blister developing or you see one appear, let us know as the dosage and type of medication may need to be changed.

### Medications

When discharged you should continue with the medicine you were taking prior to surgery to prevent a fever blister outbreak. Take these as directed until the supply is exhausted; these prescriptions need not be refilled. You will also be given several new prescriptions at the time of discharge. One of them is for the relief of pain. Sleeping pills may also be prescribed but should not be used unless you feel that you need them. An antibiotic will also be given and should be started immediately after surgery. Antibiotics should be taken until the supply is finished. They can occasionally lead to gastrointestinal upset. If this occurs notify us so your prescription can be changed.

### Depression

Because a person is so "keyed-up" before the operation, there is usually a mental and physical let-down afterward. It is not unusual for the patient to feel depressed and tired following any surgery. No matter how much they wanted the operation beforehand and how much they were informed about what to expect post-operatively, most are still surprised when they see their face swollen and discolored. Because of the initial appearance of the face following resurfacing, it is more common after this than other surgeries. If this happens do not be concerned. One looks worse for a few days following skin resurfacing as the skin swells, weeps, and crusts. Realize that every other patient experiences the same feelings. The best "treatment" is to busy one's self with postoperative care and to divert one's attention to other activities (T.V., books, etc.).

### Resuming Activities

1. Wearing Eyeglasses: If the area around the nose has been resurfaced, you should wait three (3) weeks before wearing eyeglasses for prolonged periods. The pressure of glasses resting on the skin of the nose, except for very brief periods of time, is to be avoided. When you do wear eyeglasses make sure that a piece of Saran wrap is between the skin and the eyeglasses on the bridge of your nose to prevent irritation. Do this until instructed otherwise by me.
2. Sun Exposure: Try to avoid either direct or reflected rays of the sun for at least eight (8) weeks, since increased pigmentation of the resurfaced areas may result when the new delicate skin is exposed too early. This means that sunning oneself (golfing, fishing, tennis, or similar activities) during the sunny part of the day should be avoided during the initial eight (8) week period. The resurfaced areas should be protected for six (6) months by large brimmed hats and a sun screen. I will inform you when you can utilize sun screen because if started too soon it can also irritate the new skin.
3. Returning to Work and Resuming Social Activities: When these should commence depends upon the amount of public contact, the amount of sun exposure your job involves, and the degree of redness and swelling you develop. It also depends on the depth of resurfacing with the deeper the depth taking longer to recover. The average patient returns to work or goes out socially about two (2) weeks after deep resurfacing, about 1 (1) week after medium depth resurfacing, and the same week with superficial resurfacing. Depending upon individual circumstances, social interaction can begin as soon as makeup can be worn.
4. Athletics: Strenuous athletic endeavors should be avoided for the first few weeks. Exposure to extremes of heat, cold, or wind during the early stages of healing must be avoided. Such exposure certainly causes the skin to become pink because of increased blood flow. However, this condition should subside in a short while if it occurs. Remember you should care for your new skin as carefully as that of a newborn baby. Like a baby's skin it may have a more delicate texture and possibly a different color. Your delicate new skin must toughen with time. Household cleaners, fabric softeners, lotions and creams with fragrances and preservatives, newsprint, dyes, makeups, nail polish products, astringents, detergents, hair sprays, facial tissues, or cotton balls and Q-tips, etc., could produce some irritation (contact dermatitis) during the first few weeks. Your skin will gradually toughen and tolerate most of your pre-surgical activities.

### Post-Operative Clinic Visits and Accommodations

You will be seen in the Clinic the day following your resurfacing procedure and at several intervals for the first few weeks. The exact timing of these visits will vary from individual to individual depending upon the healing process and the extent of the areas resurfaced. Please make every attempt to keep these appointments, since it is vitally important that we closely monitor your healing. Obviously, if small areas are peeled or "touched-up" the required follow up will be less and often can be done taking pictures and sending them to me for your convenience if you prefer.

### Post-Operative Instructions

Please follow these instructions carefully. Even more so than other procedures offered, your final result following resurfacing will depend upon how well you care for the treated areas and protect them from irritating materials or products. The timeline provided applies to most patients but some will heal faster and others a slower. I will provide you with specific instructions on when to proceed to the next week instructions during your follow up visits.

- KEEP HANDS AND WIPES AWAY FROM TREATED AREAS AS MUCH AS POSSIBLE. The oils and bacteria on your hands and these products can be very irritating.
- Remember your new skin is as sensitive and delicate as a newborn baby's. Don't take chances and please do not ask permission to vary from the instructions that you are given. Patients who follow them tend to heal more quickly and end up with better results.
- As healing progresses, your skin will become more resilient, but this may take 2-3 months for deep peels. Most people agree that the final results are worth the inconvenience.
- After your operation, you become the most important person in preventing problems. Please follow instructions.
- If your new skin comes in contact (directly or indirectly) with irritating substances, you might develop a rash (contact dermatitis). Should this occur, we can initiate another treatment program. But as is the case with any allergy or irritant, avoidance is the first line treatment to prevent problems.
- Tell us if you have a history of sensitive skin or other conditions such as dandruff, seborrheic dermatitis, rosacea, lupus or other collagen disorders. Patients with some of these conditions should not undergo resurfacing other than superficial treatments.
- Following your procedure, we will instruct you to use a product that has been shown to provide more comfort and to promote more rapid recovery. It is designed to provide a moist environment which promotes more rapid skin healing.

**WEEK 1 (Beginning the day after surgery)**

DO: Apply a thin coating of Aquaphor to cover areas resurfaced with lasers or dermabrasion. For peels, wait until the top layer of skin begins to shed before applying Aquaphor. This is usually around the second or third day.

DO: Keep all resurfaced areas completely covered with Aquaphor at all times. This is done to prevent drying of resurfaced areas, so that they may heal more quickly.

DO: Re-apply Aquaphor at least twice daily or as often as needed to create a protect-tive covering over the treated areas. Avoid getting Aquaphor in your eyes.

DO: Shampoo your hair the first day after surgery using CeraVe hydrating cleanser. USE ONLY THE RECOMMENDED SHAMPOO AND DO NOT USE A CONDITIONER.

DO: Avoid getting water on your face initially. A small amount is not a problem. Allow the water to air dry.

* * * * *

DO NOT: Use ANY skin care or moisturizing products anywhere on your body, except those specifically recommended by us and only when told by Dr. Guy it is okay to do so. The reason is lotion placed anywhere on the body will eventually find its way to your face inadvertently which can be irritating. Dr. Guy will instruct you on when to use CeraVe hydrating cleanser on your face and body.

DO NOT: Rub or wipe skin with Kleenex®, skin cleansers, fabrics that shed, or facial tissues at any time. We will provide you with gauzes that can be used as needed and only sparingly.

DO NOT: Use cotton balls or Q-tips® on or around the treated areas.

DO NOT: Pick at crusts as this can lead to scarring.

DO NOT: Touch your skin until after you have washed your hands thoroughly with CeraVe hydrating cleanser. Newsprint, computer paper, household cleaners, pet products and powders, detergents, cold creams, body creams, baby oil, bubble bath products, soaps that contain cold cream or fragrances, tartar control toothpaste, and toothpastes which bleach or whiten teeth should be avoided as long as any pink color remains to the new skin. All or any of these materials can cause rashes. Keep hair spray, colognes, perfumes, or any substance with a fragrance away from the treated areas at all times. As a rule, if it smells "good" or "bad" its fumes may irritate your new skin at this point. Follow the rules, protect your new skin, and you can speed up the healing process.

DO NOT: Use bleach or fabric softeners in laundry.

**WEEK 2 (after seven days)**

DO: Continue Aquaphor in week two if crusts are still present and if you are directed to do so. The objective is to soften any residual crusts. Do not use Aquaphor on skin which has no crusts as this can lead to irritation.

* * * * *

DO NOT: Use makeup during week 2 (see week three instructions).

DO NOT: Touch your skin until after you have washed your hands thoroughly with CeraVe hydrating cleanser. Refrain from handling newsprint, computer paper, household cleaners, detergents, cold creams, body creams, baby oil, bubble bath products, soaps or products that contain creams or fragrances, and tooth-paste with bleach or whitening agents. Keep hair spray, colognes, perfumes, or any other substance with a fragrance away from the treated areas at all times.

**WEEK 3**

DO: Use only mineral makeup with no sunscreen if skin is smooth and free of crusts AND if I have approved it. When makeup has been approved, please do not ask permission to use anything other than mineral makeup. Other products will be too irritating to you skin this early on.

DO: Remove makeup in the shower with water and CeraVe hydrating cleanser only.

DO: If you experience dry lips use a small amount of Aquaphor on them as instructed.

DO: Keep your hands away from the treated areas as much as possible.

* * * * *

DO NOT: Touch your skin until after you have washed your hands thoroughly with CeraVe hydrating cleanser. Refrain from handling newsprint, computer paper, household cleaners, detergents, cold creams, body creams, baby oil, bubble bath products, soaps or products that contain creams or fragrances, and toothpaste with bleach or whitening agents. Keep hair spray, colognes, perfumes, or any other substance with a fragrance away from the treated areas at all times.

**WEEK 4**

DO: Continue using CeraVe hydrating cleanser as your body wash and face wash unless instructed otherwise.

* * * * *

DO NOT: Use any other soaps, moisturizers, cleansing creams, astringents, Alpha-hydroxy acids, Retin-A, glycolic products, etc. on your face until you have been instructed to do so.

DO NOT: Touch your skin until after you have washed your hands thoroughly with CeraVe hydrating cleanser. Refrain from handling newsprint, computer paper, household cleaners, detergents, cold creams, body creams, baby oil, bubble bath products, soaps or products that contain creams or fragrances, and toothpaste with bleach or whitening agents. Keep hair spray, colognes, perfumes, or any other substance with a fragrance away from the treated areas at all times.

**WEEK 5**

DO: If the skin is not red or excessively pink, use oil-based make-up only if approved.

DO: If the skin is not red or excessively pink, begin to use your preferred skin care products. Only introduce one new product every 2 days to make sure you do not develop a rash.

DO: Use sunscreen to protect the resurfaced areas. Test a small area on your face to evaluate for the development of any redness before applying over the entire treated area. If irritation does occur do not use sunscreen until cleared by me.

DO: Resume reasonable physical activities.

* * * * *

DO NOT: Use Retin-A®, Alpha-Hydroxy acid, or "peel" products anywhere on face or body until instructed to do so.

Notify our clinic immediately if any rash or fever blister-like areas should appear.

**Remember the things you were told before your operation, namely:**

1. Swelling will increase for the first few days. It tends to swell the most around the lips and eyes. This swelling will go down.
2. The skin will begin to weep and crust. This is a normal part of the healing process. It is important to not pull off any of the crusts.
3. Continue to use the Aquaphor over the resurfaced areas until instructed other-wise. This is done to help soften the crusts.
4. Avoid touching your face with any items as it can lead to a rash in the immediate post treatment period.
5. Only use the CeraVe hydrating cleanser as both the shampoo and body cleanser once instructed by us.
6. Healing takes time. The results of skin resurfacing depend on following the instructions more so than any other surgical procedure.

7. The answer to most questions about "When can I . . ." is "When the pink goes away." Starting to use products too soon can lead to prolonged pink skin.
8. Most of all, BE PATIENT during the healing process. It truly is a process. If you have further questions, you are urged to call us and keep your appointments.

**Report to the Clinic Any:**

1. Temperature elevation greater than 100 degrees
2. Sudden swelling or discoloration.
3. Hemorrhage.
4. Discharge from the wound edges or other evidence of infection.
5. Development of any reaction to medications.

If you have any questions call 832-956-1040

# Chapter 13

## Scar Revision Surgery

**Scar Revision and Skin Surgery**

**Scar Healing**

**Stages of Reconstruction**

**After Scar Revision**

*Post-Operative Instructions*
*Remember the things you were told before your operation, namely*
*Report to the Clinic Any*

# Scar Revision and Skin Surgery

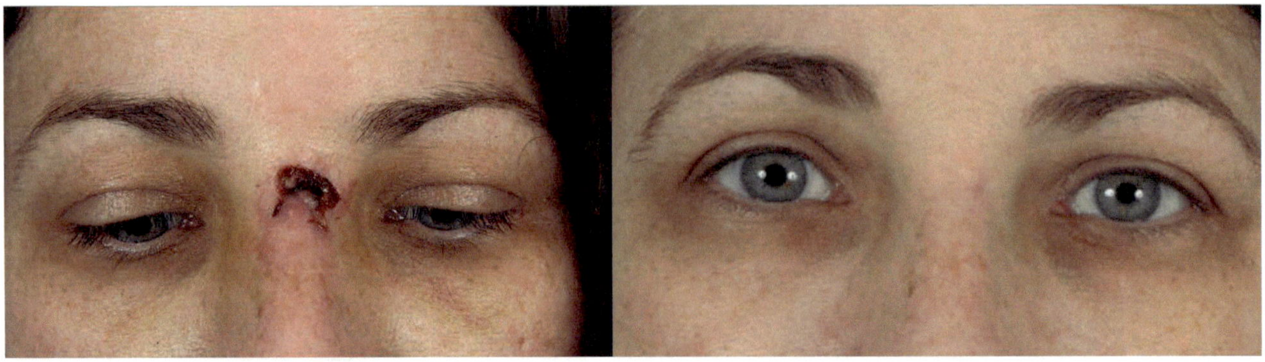

Before After

The above patient presented with the before scar following a trauma. After local wound care was initiated, her scar was both depressed and irregular. She underwent excision of her scar followed by CO2 laser which left her with the after scar you see above.

Unsightly, disfiguring scars, or skin defects can be disconcerting and often devastating to one's self-image. In addition to scars, other blemishes or defects that may be removed or improved with carefully planned plastic surgery techniques include moles, skin cancers, cysts, and other bumps.

These lesions may be partially or completely excised with surgery. However, a defect will result which must be repaired. Repair options include advancing the edges together (primary closure), allowing the wound to heal on its own (rarely performed), skin grafts, or flaps from adjacent skin. Each incision made into the skin, regardless of where it is placed, who makes it, for what purpose it is made, or whether it is deliberate or accidental heals by producing a scar. This simple fact is frequently forgotten or ignored by individuals who think that a "plastic surgeon" can make an incision and leave no visible scar and that he can eliminate existing scars.

The appearance of most scars or blemishes may be improved by well-planned and carefully executed surgery, but there are some important facts patients contemplating such procedures should know.

Scars are usually unsightly because they may:

- Be wide
- Be longer than one inch
- Cross natural creases or facial contour lines
- Be elevated above the adjacent skin
- Be depressed below the adjacent skin
- Be a different color than adjacent tissues
- Distort other facial features

If any or all of these characteristics are present, improvement in any one of them should make the scar(s) less conspicuous. Correction of two or three of these factors can often result in dramatic improvement of the appearance (and sometimes function) of the scar(s). By using plastic surgery techniques, I can lead to the most favorable scar. Attempts are made to place incisions in the least conspicuous place possible for improved cosmetics. With scar revision, the surgeon's goal is to replace an unsightly or disfiguring scar with a better scar. The final appearance however is dependent on many factors, one of which is the patient's own healing capability. In most situations, additional revision surgery including resurfacing can help provide an improved result, especially in the case of skin cancer repair.

## Scar Healing

Possibly conditioned by what they see on television and in the movies, many people expect the final result immediately and become disappointed and troubled because they have to wait for "maturation" of their scars. Maturation is the continuing change in appearance all scars go through until they reach a state where no further change will occur. Maturation of scars may take from 6 to 18 months, and sometimes longer in young children. Initially, a freshly repaired incision or scar usually looks very good. Then it becomes reddened, possibly somewhat raised above the surrounding skin, and frequently is hard or lumpy. This is the body laying down healing tissue. Unless the scar is frequently stressed by stretching the surrounding skin, the firmness and red color lessen and should disappear gradually. This leaves a softer scar which is usually more level with and somewhat lighter in color than the adjacent skin.

Patients seeking scar revision should be emotionally prepared to accept several facts: First, removal will result in another, though hopefully, improved scar; second, the final appearance will not be evident for 6 to 18 months; and third, more than one procedure is usually required as scar revision is a process.

This brings us to another very important matter. Understandably, most people with recent scarring want repair immediately. However, scar revision, except in selected cases, should not be undertaken too soon. The passage of time is the best, the kindest, and, in the long run, the simplest treatment to give to any scar of recent origin. The reason is that most scars will undergo spontaneous improvement if given enough time to do so.

Only after the scar has become soft and white is it "mature." A decision regarding a second stage revision may be delayed until this time has elapsed. However, scars which cause distortion of normal structures (eyebrows, lips, eyelids, nostrils, etc.) those which spread widely or produce deformity by contraction, and "U" or "J" shaped scars may be repaired earlier because little or no improvement in the basic problem can be anticipated with the passage of time.

When removing an existing scar or blemish by excision, I make every effort to place the line of incision as nearly as possible in or parallel to one of the normal crease lines of the face or body. This helps to camouflage the scar. Sometimes it may be necessary to change the direction of a scar so that it will follow these lines. Excision of large unsightly scars, birthmarks, or blemishes may require multiple operations over a period of time (called serial excision). This takes advantage of the skin's natural ability to stretch which allows more normal skin to be used to close the large defect. Occasionally, it is necessary to shift surrounding tissue to fill a defect, or rarely, even resort to skin grafting.

## Stages of Reconstruction

Scar revision often requires at least two and frequently three surgical procedures to obtain the best achievable result. Usually 3-6 months separate each stage, although when lasers and dermabrasion are used, they may be performed more quickly. Some scars "mature" more quickly, and subsequent stages may be performed sooner. One of the paradoxes of healing is that scars on younger children may take 18-24 months, sometimes longer, to mature, while the same scar on a patient in their 60's may be flat, thin, and soft within 3 months. This is one of the unpredictable factors that accounts for the variability in the final result that occurs with scar revision and wound healing. Since resurfacing with lasers or dermabrasion is usually a vital part of most scar revisions, you should read the section on resurfacing carefully (page 98).

## After Scar Revision

The following are designed to answer practically every question that may arise regarding the "do's" and "don'ts" after surgery. You and your family should read the instructions several times to familiarize yourselves thoroughly with them. Attempt to follow them faithfully, because those who do so generally have the smoothest post-operative course. This, of course, favors proper healing and a better result. Failure to follow these instructions faithfully can lead to certain complications which potentially could jeopardize the desired result.

Whenever a question arises, refer back to this book. Chances are you will find the answer, but if you cannot please call us (832-956-1040). If you ever have a concern, call us. It is essential that our staff has the opportunity to evaluate any problem which may arise.

### Post-Operative Instructions

When incisions have been made into the skin to remove existing scars or blemishes, the new skin edges are carefully approximated with fine delicate sutures (metal clips in the hair bearing scalp). It takes several days for the wound edges to mend so the immediate post-operative period is crucial in your getting the best possible result. Be careful not to injure the surgical area. Some swelling and discoloration can be expected with any surgical procedure. It can be minimized by applying cold compresses over the operated area during the first 48 to 72 hours, but never place anything directly from the freezer on your skin.

The swelling is due to the new tissue fluids brought into the area by the body to promote healing. The increased blood supply to the region is responsible for the pink color of the skin and some of the "discoloration" associated with surgery. When these healing fluids are no longer required, the tissues release them and they are absorbed through the bloodstream.

You must be willing to accept temporary swelling and discoloration which occurs following such operations. Though usually visually disconcerting, most people feel it is a negligible inconvenience to pay for the physical and psychological improvement they generally experience.

In many situations, a tape dressing is placed over the suture line to help protect it. Do not disturb the tapes and try not to get them wet. They will be removed during your one-week post-operative visit. Often the incision sites may be re-taped for an additional week to allow for further healing when possible.

We sometimes use a dissolvable suture to close surgical incisions. When the tape dressing is placed over them, the surface suture material ordinarily comes off when the tape is removed. More often, permanent sutures are used. Any permanent sutures and any remaining dissolvable sutures are removed around one week with delicate instruments.

When the incisions have been placed in areas where tape would not stick to the skin (on the lip margin or around the eyelid), tape is not applied over the sutures, so close adherence to the following instructions is essential.

When no tape has been placed over the suture line, we recommend you follow this routine. Six times daily you should:

1. Saturate a Q-tip with full strength hydrogen peroxide.
2. Gently roll over the suture line with the peroxide moistened Q-tip by to help dissolve any crusts. This is not a rubbing over the suture line which could damage the sutures but rather a gentle motion. You are not expected to remove all crusts at each cleaning.
3. Always move the Q-tip along (parallel to) the suture line and never across (perpendicular) to it as this could pop a suture and lead to unfavorable healing.
4. Following each peroxide treatment apply a thin layer of the recommended ointment to the suture line. The recommended ointment is usually bacitracin or Aquaphor as they have a low chance of causing skin irritation. Keeping the wound moist like this improves and speeds wound healing.

We will usually recommend you continue this treatment program for as long as there is any crusting along the suture line. As the crusting decreases you can decrease the frequency of cleaning, although the wound should still be covered with ointment to keep it moist.

In most patients, makeup may be applied to the surgical area for camouflaging within 2-3 days after the tapes or sutures are removed (about 10 days after the original surgery). Apply and remove it carefully as any excessive force can delay healing and lead to a worse scar.

Once the crusting is gone, the use of a silicone-based gel is usually recommended. Studies have only shown silicone to have a positive impact on the appearance of scars. Vitamin E products like Mederma® have not been shown to improve scars in clinical studies and is not recommended.

**Remember the things you were told before your operation, namely:**

1. It takes time (6-12 months) for the scar to mature. It will get red and lumpy before it begins to flatten and become lighter in color. Not until it is white and flat is it mature, so be patient. Sometimes steroid injections every 3-4 weeks can reduce excessive lumpiness and speed healing if it is needed.
2. In most scar revision cases, more than one operation will be necessary in order to obtain the best possible result. The first procedure generally requires excisional surgery with suture repair. Later stages usually require dermabrasion or lasers so read these sections carefully (Pages 102 and 105).
3. We will advise you as to when your next stage should be performed.
4. Notify us if you suspect any problem such as infection, undue swelling, or

redness, or if the sutures come out prematurely.

5. Notify us if you are unsure about the instructions you are to follow as they are important in attaining the best cosmetic result.
6. Failure to follow these instructions faithfully can lead to certain complications which potentially could jeopardize the desired result.

**Report to the Clinic Any:**

1. Temperature elevation greater than 100 degrees
2. Sudden swelling or discoloration.
3. Hemorrhage.
4. Discharge from the wound edges or other evidence of infection.
5. Development of any reaction to medications.

If you have any questions call

832-956-1040

# CHAPTER 14

## Skin Cancer

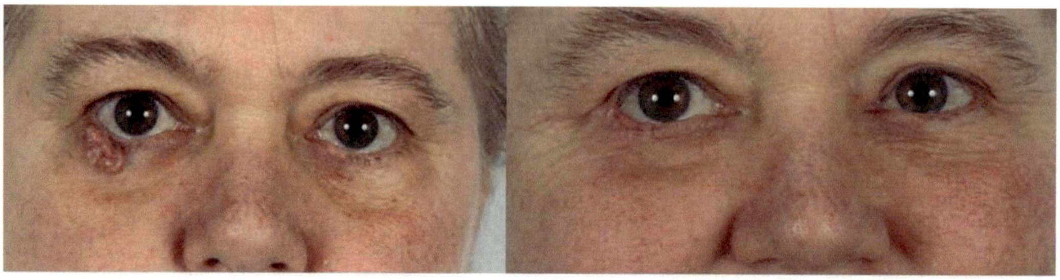

Before After

This patient underwent a skin cancer removal from below her right eyelid. As you can see Dr. Guy is skilled in both the removal and reconstruction. This patient 8 weeks out from her surgery shows a very natural appearance of her eyelid following the repair of a defect that involved all layers of her eyelid.

## Types of Skin Cancers

Skin cancer is the most common type of cancer in the United States and is directly linked to ultraviolet (UV) exposure. This may be from the sun or from tanning beds. One in five Americans will develop some form of skin cancer over his or her lifetime. Any sun burn increases your chance of developing these types of cancers, and the effects are cumulative. Certain people are more predisposed to developing skin cancer including those with light hair, blue eyes, and fair skin. Those who are immune-suppressed, whether from transplants or other cancer treatments are also at a higher risk. The three most common types are basal cell carcinoma, squamous cell carcinoma, and melanoma, in that order.

Concerning findings include any skin lesion that is growing, becoming itchy, or bleeds and never seems to heal. Basal cell carcinoma is the most common but least aggressive. It tends to develop around the nose and ears but it can be found anywhere on the face. It grows slowly and has almost no chance of spreading, although it can become locally destructive if not treated in a timely fashion. Treatment options include freezing them (cryotherapy), shaving them (curettage), radiation (rarely used), topical medications, and surgery. Factors that help decide the best treatment option include your overall health, history of previous skin cancers, and previous treatments you have received as recurrent cancers tend to be more aggressive.

Squamous cell carcinoma is the next most common. It can develop anywhere on the face, but sun exposed areas such as the ears and scalp may have a higher likelihood of having squamous cell carcinomas. It can also be found in long standing scars or ulcers. This type of skin cancer grows faster than basal cell carcinoma. If not addressed early enough, it does have a chance of spreading. Treatment most commonly involves surgery but for select, early lesions, some topical creams can be used. Radiation is also an option in very specific circumstances.

Melanoma is the least common of the three but is the most aggressive and increasing in incidence in the United States. Even small lesions can spread early. The

ABC's of melanoma include Asymmetry or that the lesion is not circular, Borders that are uneven or irregular, multiple Colors (brown, black, and red), a Diameter larger than a pencil eraser, and finally Evolving or changing in size, shape, or color. Treatment involves surgery and may involve other therapy depending on the stage.

If you have any moles or skin growths that you are concerned about, it is best to have your dermatologist examine these. Any growth that is suspicious should be biopsied to rule out the possibility of a cancer. Remember, if treated early, almost all skin cancers are curable.

## Skin Cancer Treatment

There are several ways of surgically removing skin cancers. The following include a description of the options available in the treatment of non-melanoma skin cancer. Depending on the size and location of the skin cancer, the health of the patient, and the desires of the patient, one treatment option may be better than another. I am skilled in both the cancer removal (other than Mohs' surgery) as well as the reconstructive techniques in order to give you the most aesthetically pleasing scar and get you back to your normal activities, cancer free.

### Mohs' Micrographic Surgery

Mohs' surgery is a modified form of surgical excision that provides for an accurate assessment of the completeness of tumor removal with a very high cure rate and may be more tissue-sparing than conventional surgery. It involves the Mohs' surgeon taking a small amount of tissue around the tumor. The surgeon is then the one that processes the tissue and looks at it under the microscope. This method provides for an almost complete evaluation of all of the edges of the tumor microscopically to verify it has been removed. This leads to an almost 99% cure rate for early basal cell cancers. It does require special training by the surgeon to enable him or her to microscopically evaluate the excised tissue. As a result, this type of surgery requires special equipment and can be more expensive and time-consuming than conventional surgery. Thus, Mohs' surgery is usually reserved for those instances where it is very important to preserve normal skin (i.e., eyes, nose, lips, ears, etc.) or where other types of treatments have either failed or would not be as successful.

### Electrodesiccation and Curettage (ED&C)

A form of destruction of the cancer essentially consisting of scraping (curettage) and burning with electrical current (electrodesiccating) the visible and palpable tumor and some surrounding skin. This method is based on the fact that skin cancers are softer than the surrounding normal tissue and the heat from the electric current kills the remaining cells. This procedure does not provide a method of assessing whether the tumor is completely destroyed. It usually results in a circular wound that heals with a circular scar in 3-8 weeks with local wound care. It should be used only to treat primary (never treated) skin cancer and only ones that are superficial. Since there is no assessment of whether all of the tumor has been removed this method has a higher rate of recurrence than other methods.

### Cryosurgery

This treatment method involves destroying the skin cancer cells utilizing intense cold in the form of liquid nitrogen. Like ED&C, this method does not provide for assessment of complete tumor destruction and has the same limitations as ED&C. It usually heals similarly to ED&C leaving a circular scar.

### Surgical Excision

This method provides for the removal of a skin cancer and subsequent repair of the wound thus created. It provides tissue for microscopic assessment of the completeness of tumor removal. However, using the usual laboratory tissue processing techniques this assessment of tumor removal, although good, is not as complete as with Mohs' surgery. However, by taking an appropriate healthy cuff of normal tissue around the tumor based on research it also provides for a very high cure rate close to 95%. Surgical excision usually heals in 1-2 weeks with a linear or geometric scar depending on the extent of surgery required. However, some patients, depending on the nature of their tumor, could require extensive reconstruct-tion. After the scars are mature additional plastic surgical techniques may be used to improve and/or camouflage them. Surgery for skin cancers is usually performed under local anesthesia as an outpatient.

### Radiation Therapy

A form of destruction of the skin cancer utilizing radiation energy. It is useful in those patients that are not healthy enough to toler-ate a surgical procedure or those with a lot of sun damage who are developing multiple skin cancers. It can be used to treat primary tumors; however, it does not provide assessment of the completeness of tumor destruction. Healing takes place over 4-8 weeks, usually with a good cosmetic response. However, some patients can develop significant scarring and radiation damage of the skin with many long-term complications, so it is not usually performed on younger patients. Occasionally the radiation can result many years later in the development of a new skin cancer in the area of previous treatment. Radiation therapy is usually performed over a period of 3-5 weeks.

### Topical Treatment

For early skin cancers or premalignant skin lesions, there are topical medications available. These tend to cause the skin to become red and blister which is what helps to remove the superficial skin lesions. Deeper chemical peeling agents can also be used on premalignant lesions but not on true skin cancers. The therapy is continued over several weeks during which time the skin does become quite raw, but the healing is usually without a scar.

## Skin Cancer Surgery

The following is meant to provide you with an overview of what to expect if you choose the surgical route for treatment. It includes information regarding before, during, and after surgery. It should help to provide you at ease for the process.

### What is the Purpose of the Pre-Operative or Initial Visit?

The initial visit allows Dr. Guy the opportu-nity to examine your skin lesion, obtain your medical history, and biopsy the lesion, if necessary, in order to determine the best way of treating your skin cancer. At that time, the method of treatment, pre-operative instructions, the need for possible hospital-ization, and the need for adjustments in any of your medications will be deter-mined. When patients are referred to Dr. Guy by other physicians, a biopsy and pathology report stating the type of skin cancer is usually available. If this is not available, a biopsy will be necessary since all skin cancers are not alike. It is necessary to know the type of skin cancer you have before we can choose the best method of treatment.

### Getting Ready for Surgery

It is advisable that you get a good night's sleep. Please do not take aspirin or aspirin-containing products or other over-the-counter pain medications other than Tylenol ® for two weeks prior to the surgery, since these medications cause more bleeding. Also, please do not drink alcoholic beverages for three days prior to your surgery since alcohol dilates blood vessels and aggravates bleeding problems. Smoking may impair your healing and should be stopped at least seventy-two (72) hours before and after surgery to promote wound healing. Continue all your regular medicines unless you are instructed otherwise.

If you will undergo Mohs' surgery, be sure to follow the instructions provided by the Mohs' surgeon. It is a good idea to bring a book or magazine on the day of Mohs' surgery since the procedure may take a full day with a lot of waiting for the skin to be checked for cancer. Also, it is recommended that you bring a person with you that can provide company in the waiting room and drive you home, as well as assist you at home after the surgery.

### The Day of Surgery

When you arrive for reconstructive surgery, Dr. Guy will answer any questions that may remain. You will then be asked to sign a consent form, and we will obtain pictures (when appropriate) of the acquired skin defect for the medical record and teaching purposes. The surgical site will be prepared and the surgery will proceed as planned. Afterwards the doctor and/or assistant will bandage the surgical area and review post-operative wound instructions.

Mohs' surgery cases are usually scheduled early in the day. The surgery is usually performed in stages and, in some cases, can last the entire day. In these cases, you may not be following up with us until the following day. Surgical repair is usually performed in the afternoon after the Mohs' surgery is completed or sometimes later in the week.

### The Surgical Wound

When the skin cancer is completely removed, a decision is then made with regard to the appropriate method for treating the wound which has been created. The usual choices include:

1. Letting the wound heal by itself (secondary intention)
2. Closing the wound with stitches (primary closure)
3. Closing the wound with a skin graft from another part of the body
4. Closing the wound with adjacent skin
5. Closing the wound with skin that is close but not adjacent

The method used will be determined by the nature, extent, and location of the tumor and the resultant wound. It also depends on your overall health. We will recommend which of these methods is best suited in your case. Attempts will be made to describe the repair that is likely before you undergo Mohs' surgery but at times, especially with recurrent tumors, the tissue removed is larger than what was originally expected. However, the treatment plan is always discussed with the patient before proceeding with it.

## After Skin Cancer Surgery

If the wound is allowed to heal by itself it usually heals over 4-8 weeks depending on its size. If the other methods, except delayed closure, are used, it usually heals in 1-2 weeks. All wounds normally drain a yellowish, amber color, and dressings need to be changed with each cleansing to prevent crust formation. Under no circumstances should the wound be immersed under water, as in a bathtub, pool, or spa, but showering is acceptable.

All wounds can initially be faintly red, slightly tender, itch, drain amber fluid, and show some swelling that disappears gradually. However, persistence or an increase in these signs and symptoms may indicate a problem such as infection and should be brought to the doctor's attention.

### What if I Don't Like the Scar?

If you find the final scar to be unsatisfactory, there are various treatments that can be attempted in order to modify the scar (See chapter 13 Scar Revision Surgery). In any event, we recommend that you wait at least 5 weeks before seeking modification of a scar, since scars undergo their own biological modification. Even then, the recommendation may be to wait longer depending on how the scar is healing. Dermabrasion and lasers can be performed to modify the scar and is ideally performed 6 weeks after surgery if needed. It may take 12-18 months for scars to mature, so be patient.

### Follow-Up Surgery?

A follow-up period of at least five years is necessary after the wound has healed. Experience has shown that recurrence of the skin cancer usually occurs within the first year of surgery and that once you develop a skin cancer there is a 50% chance you will develop others. Thus, you will be asked to return for follow-up of the surgical site and for a skin examinations by your dermatologist routinely and more commonly in the first year. If you were referred by another physician this follow-up can be performed by him or her. Any suspicious area should be evaluated at once.

### What About Exposure to the Sun?

The damage from the sun is cumulative. It is helpful to prevent any further damage with the use of sunscreen and physical blockers such as hats and clothing. It is recommended you use at least an SPF 30 sunscreen, and reapply often if you need to be out in the sun. If you perspire or swim, you should reapply it liberally. In addition, avoiding the hours of sun between 10:00 A.M. and 4:00 P.M. can further help protect you as this is when the sun's rays are the most direct and damaging.

### Post-Operative Instructions

The wound should be kept absolutely clean and dry for the first day. If there is not an overlying bandage, the wound should be cleaned gently with hydrogen peroxide on a Q-tip at least six (6) times daily. The recommended antibacterial ointment should be applied after each cleaning to the incision line. Suture removal will usually be in 1 to 2 weeks depending on the extent of the wound.

Most patients do not complain of pain. However, if you are uncomfortable, we recommend taking Tylenol® (acetaminophen) as directed but do not take any other over-the-counter pain relievers as they thin the blood. If this fails to provide relief then take the prescribed pain medication as needed.

Uncommonly, there may be continued bleeding following surgery. It is normal to have a small amount of blood on the bandages, but if it is more than this or a continuous flow, lie down, remove all bandages, and with sterile gauze apply firm pressure continuously for 20-30 minutes at the site of bleeding. If the bleeding appears brisk, also notify our office (832-956-1040) as you undergo this maneuver. If bleeding stops, do not remove the bandages as this may dislodge a clot and restart the bleeding. Secure the bandage with tape and see us in the office as soon as possible. If the bleeding persists after 20-30 minutes notify our office or call 832-956-1040 to reach the doctor. If you cannot reach the doctor, go to the nearest hospital or Emergency Room.

Please follow these instructions carefully as they have been created to help you achieve the best functional and cosmetic result.

1. Do not shower for 24 hours after the procedure.
2. If the wound is bandaged, leave it that way. Avoid touching the area and do not get the bandages wet.
3. If the wound is not bandaged, clean it gently at least six (6) times daily with hydrogen peroxide on a Q-tip. Following cleaning apply the recommended antibiotic ointment to the area to help with healing.
4. If the wound is not bandaged, it is okay to have a shower daily after 24 hours but do not ever submerge the wound under water as in bathing or swimming until instructed it is okay.

After the wound heals, you may notice a red scar that gradually fades. The scar can be elevated or depressed initially, but usually flattens. Sometimes the scar can be sensitive to touch or temperature or can have altered sensations such as itching or numbness, which usually improve with time. Rarely, some of these changes may be permanent.

**Remember the things you were told before your operation, namely:**

Skin cancer when treated early has a high cure rate. It also requires less skin to be removed and can allow for more readily performed reconstruction.

It is important to have regular follow up after any skin cancer has been removed. There is a 50% chance of developing a second skin cancer so routine skin checks are needed.

For more advanced skin cancers, the reconstruction may require multiple stages. This would be discussed with you prior to the surgery as it does require local wound care between stages, and in some cases can leave a visually disconcerting wound until the final stage is undertaken.

It takes time (6-12 months) for the scar to mature. It will get red and lumpy before it begins to flatten and become lighter in color. Not until it is white and flat is it mature, so be patient. Sometimes steroid injections every 3-4 weeks can reduce excessive lumpiness and speed healing if it is needed.

Notify us if you suspect any problem such as infection, undue swelling, or redness, or if the sutures come out prematurely.

**Report to the Clinic Any:**

1. Temperature elevation greater than 100 degrees
2. Sudden swelling or discoloration.
3. Hemorrhage.
4. Discharge from the wound edges or other evidence of infection.
5. Development of any reaction to medications.

If you have any questions call
832-956-1040

# Chapter 15

## Neuromodulators (Botox, Dysport, and Daxxify) and Fillers

## Neuromodulators

Botox was the first product developed in a line of treatments known as neuromodulators. It has been used since the 1970s for various medical conditions in the head and neck including migraine headaches, difficulty swallowing (dysphagia), excessive sweating, sweating when eating, problems with the voice, and eye twitching. It works by inhibiting the action of muscles. This can be used to your advantage by selectively inhibiting muscles that cause wrinkles. Common locations for its use include the forehead, the area between the eyes (glabella), the areas next to the eyes (crow's feet or lateral orbital rhytids), the bands of the neck (platysmal bands), and the mid portion of the nose (bunny lines). Other areas it can be used include to soften the fine wrinkles around the mouth, the dimples of the chin, and thc muscles that cause frowns (depressor anguli oris) in order to help turn up the corners of the mouth.

There are several drugs in the same class as Botox including Dysport, Xeomin, Jeuveau, and Daxxify. Each manufacturer determines what a "unit" is, and there is not a comparable relationship between unit amounts required for each treatment area. In other words, 1 unit of Botox is not the same as 1 unit of Dysport. Whereas neuromodulators can be very helpful for the right patient, it is not for everyone. It can also be used to help improve the results of more invasive treatments such as surgery or skin resurfacing.

It is important to realize that neuromodulators take time to work. Although some patients will "feel" an effect later that evening, most patients will begin to notice an effect in about 3 days, reaching a maximum effect in 7-14 days, and lasting for about 3 months. Daxxify tends to last the longest with benefits up to 6-9 months for over half of patients, but this is not to be expected in everyone.

## Fillers

Fillers work differently from neuromodulators. They are a group of products that are less invasive than surgery and used to augment the soft tissues of the face. They can help to smooth out lines and creases. They can fill out depressed scars. They can help to restore volume which has become ptotic (droopy) with aging.

Common locations to use fillers include the deep creases areas around the mouth (melolabial folds, marionette lines), the fine wrinkles around the mouth, adding volume to the lips, and improving the fullness of the cheeks.

There are many different types of filler material. The original fillers involved using collagen derived from cows. The problem is that about 5-10% of people would have an allergic reaction and they did not last that long. A novel approach was using the cells in your own body to create new collagen. This helped to eliminate the risk of a reaction but as you can imagine, it was difficult to harvest the cells, grow them in a laboratory, have the collagen sent back, and then inject it. This also was not permanent so more permanent options were developed. The problem, in my opinion, with permanent fillers is just that, they are permanent. Your body will continue to age and what looks good at the time of augmentation may not look good in 10 years as the surrounding tissue ages. This included options like Silicone and Bellafill. Working with these fillers led to the development of some of the more commonly used and safest HA (hyaluronic acid) fillers. This is a material that is found naturally in the body and with new purer formulations since the year 2000, they have almost eliminated the risk of a local reaction. They are not permanent, but the lifespan of the fillers has improved from a few months to a few years depending on the filler chosen. The different characteristics of the various HA fillers affects how smooth they feel, where they can be injected, and how long they last.

My philosophy with fillers is to be conservative. The goal is to create a very nice but natural look. I am not a fan of fake, blown-up faces and lips, and I will not give you this result. Although there is an injectable material that can be given to get rid of the product if you aren't pleased, it is rare that we are asked to dissolve filler we injected. It is important to realize it takes up to two weeks to see the final result with fillers. Because of this, if you need more it is quite easy to add just a little extra at that time, but give it time to avoid being "overdone" with the initial injection.

## Treatment

With the use of neuromodulators or fillers, very small needles are required to introduce the material. I employ multiple methods to make this as pleasant of an experience as possible. First, ice packs are used to help numb your skin for any procedure. If you are also undergoing a filler procedure, a topical numbing medication is used. Finally, I have a gentle touch and on multiple occasions have been told "that was the easiest treatment I have ever had."

I prefer to take my time with the injections, unless you are in a hurry. This allows for a great opportunity to get to know each other. The extra time is also designed to help minimize any bruising which is possible with any injectables. If you are able to not take any blood thinners such as aspirin, ibuprofen, Plavix, Coumadin, Warfarin, etc. for one week prior to the injections your chance of developing a bruise significantly drops. With the techniques I use as well as the use of the AccuVein vein finder it is not common for patients to develop any significant bruising. Most patients feel they are a small price to pay for the results achieved.

## After Treatment

*Botox/Dysport/Daxxify*: Small units of neuromodulators have been placed into very precise areas. If you engage in activities that cause it to move, you can affect your result in a negative way. For this reason, it is important:

- Not to rub or massage the areas that received treatment for 24 hours.
- Avoid bending over or doing any activity where your head is below your heart for 4 hours. This includes avoiding lying down.
- Finally, avoid any exercise for the remainder of the day as this would increase your heart rate and blood pressure and with the increased blood flow to the face could move the neuromodulator.

By following these simple instructions, you can significantly decrease the risk of the neuromodulators spreading to unwanted areas and have an improved cosmetic outcome.

*Fillers*: Fillers are placed in larger quantities under the skin when compared with Botox. Because of this, you can feel the product initially. This sensation will decrease. With fillers as opposed to Botox, you will also see an immediate result. And the product acts like a sponge sucking up water from the body which helps to improve the result. Because of this, I say if you like it on the day of injection you will love it in two weeks. After that time, if you need a little touch up then more could be added. In order to get the best result possible and prevent the development of lumps, I recommend my rule of 3:

- Massage the injected areas as shown on the day of Injection for 30 seconds, 3 times per day, for 3 days.

It is important to realize that this is a gentle massage. You are not trying to push the filler away because if you push too hard two things can happen: First, you can bruise yourself, and second, you actually can move the filler for the first week into areas that we didn't want to fill.

It is important to realize with any injectables that these are procedures and they carry risks, however small they may be. These will be discussed on the day of your injection prior to your signing the forms consenting to the procedure. If you have any questions, please ask them before agreeing to treatment.

**Report to the clinic any:**

1. Darkening of your overlying skin in the area of injections that is more than a bruise
2. Persistent lumpiness of the filler injection
3. Redness or swelling around the injection sites
4. Anything that concerns you

If you have any questions call

832-956-1040

# Chapter 16

# Patient's Bill of Rights

# A Patient's Bill of Rights

Dr. Guy Facial Plastic Surgery (Dr. Guy FPS) publishes the following Patient's Bill of Rights to affirm its dedication to the deliverance of quality medical care. It further affirms that patients are entitled to such rights regardless of sex, cultural, economic, educational, or religious background, or the source of payment for their care. All such rights also apply to the person who may have legal responsibility to make decisions regarding medical care on behalf of the patient.

**Accordingly, all patients of Dr. Guy FPS have the right:**

1. To considerate and respectful medical care and dignity.
2. To actively participate in decisions regarding one's care and to receive as much information as is necessary to give informed consent. This includes one's right to be told before an operation, in language one can reasonably be expected to understand, the diagnosis of one's condition and the treatment being recommended, with a description of that treatment, the goal of the operation or treatment, its risks and limitations, the morbidity that usually ensues, and alternative methods of treatment. In addition, one will be given an opportunity to ask questions and have one's questions answered in a direct and straightforward manner.
3. To considerate, respectful care and services at all times and under all circumstances. This includes recognition of psychosocial, spiritual, and cultural variables that may influence the perception of your illness.
4. To refuse treatment and to be informed of the medical consequences of that action.
5. To expect privacy, discreetness, and confidentiality relative to all dealings with Dr. Guy FPS.
6. To receive pertinent instructions regarding post-operative care and appointments.
7. To receive reasonable responses in a timely fashion to any reasonable request one makes for service.
8. To reasonable continuity of care by the doctor and/or the doctor's staff, and to be informed in advance of the time and location of that care.
9. To be advised if Dr. Guy proposes to engage in or perform medical research which may affect one's care or treatment, and a right to participate or refuse to participate in such research projects.
10. To examine and receive an explanation of charges and insurance reimbursements regardless of the source of payment.
11. To express grievances and suggestions, preferably in writing, to the Administrator.
12. To be informed that one may change physicians if desired.

**Accordingly, all patients of Dr. Guy FPS have the responsibility to:**

1. Give accurate and complete health information concerning your past and current illnesses, hospitalizations, medications, allergies, and other pertinent items.

2. Assist in maintaining a safe environment.
3. Inform the physician or staff when one will not be able to keep a medical visit.
4. Participate in the development of one's care. You are responsible for your actions if you do not follow the physician's instructions. If you cannot follow through with the prescribed treatment plan, you are responsible for informing the physician.
5. Adhere to your developed care plan.
6. Request further information concerning anything one does not understand.
7. Give information regarding concerns and problems one has to the Administrator of the facility.
8. Give the staff an opportunity to try to resolve any grievance which might arise as a result of treatment.
9. Comply with recommendations for or against treatment if in the opinion of Dr. Guy, the services requested could jeopardize the health, welfare and well-being of the patient or prospective patient.
10. Have realistic expectations regarding what can be achieved with surgical and non-surgical cosmetic treatments.
11. You are responsible for ensuring that the financial obligations of health care services are fulfilled as promptly as possible and for providing up-to-date insurance information.
13. You are responsible for being considerate of the rights of other patients and personnel and for assisting in the control of noise, smoking, and the number of visitors. You also are responsible for being respectful of practice property and property of other persons visiting the practice.
14. Be responsible for lifestyle choices. Your health depends not just on the care provided at this facility but on the long-term decisions you make in daily life. You are responsible for recognizing the effects of these decisions on your health.

# NOTES

Made in the USA
Las Vegas, NV
03 November 2026

57423449R00083